T0072146

Advance Praise for
What Happened to Moderation?

"Finally, a common-sense health manual for the rest of us—the folks who aren't triathletes, fanatic calorie counters, or fad followers. Just people trying to live a healthy life making everyday decisions about what to eat and the best way to exercise and take care of ourselves and those we love. Written by a wise doctor with decades of experience caring for thousands of patients from all walks of life, this honest book lays out a core message with real promise: Extremism in the pursuit of health is no virtue; moderation is the better answer."

> **—John Danner,** *Wall Street Journal* bestselling author, university faculty member, MPH

"In a world full of fad diets, exercise cults, and abundant media stories about the latest health risks, Dr. Brewer's common-sense approach to health and wellness is a much needed source of reliable medical information. The recommendations are scientifically sound and clearly explained to guide the reader on a safe and well-balanced path to healthy living."

> **—Lee Schwamm, MD, FAHA, FANA,** Executive Vice Chairman of Neurology at Massachusetts General Hospital and Professor of Neurology at Harvard Medical School

"Dr. Brewer, a physician with a ton of medical experience, provides very practical and sound advice in an era loaded with extreme and confusing fads.

> **—John C. Goff,** Founder and Chairman of Goff Capital and Crescent Real Estate, Chairman and owner of Canyon Ranch

What Happened to Moderation?

OTHER BOOKS BY THIS AUTHOR

The Canyon Ranch Guide to Men's Health:
A Doctor's Prescription for Male Wellness
(2016)

The Everest Principle: How to Achieve the Summit of Your Life
Coauthored with Peggy Holt Wagner, MS, LPC
(2010)

What Happened to Moderation?

A Common-Sense Approach
to Improving Our Health and
Treating Common Illnesses
in an Age of Extremes

Stephen C. Brewer, MD, ABFM

Medical Director, Canyon Ranch Wellness Resorts
Tucson, Arizona

SelectBooks, Inc.
New York

This material has been written and published for educational purposes to enhance one's well-being in regard to health issues and physical fitness. The information contained herein presents the viewpoint of the author and is not necessarily that of the publisher. This information given by the author is not intended for the diagnosis of any medical condition, and the material presented here is not intended to be a substitute for an individual's prescribed medications, prescribed exercise program, special diet recommendations, or psychiatric or psychological treatments or therapies. Consult with your primary care physician before engaging in any new exercise program or change in diet.

Reliance on any information provided herein is at your own risk. The publisher and author will have no responsibility to any person or entity with respect to loss, damage, or injury claimed to be caused directly or indirectly by any information in this book.

Copyright © 2019 by Stephen C. Brewer

All rights reserved. Published in the United States of America. No part of this book may be reproduced or transmitted in any form or by any means, graphic, electronic, or mechanical, including photocopying, recording, taping or by any information storage or retrieval system, without the permission in writing from the publisher.

This edition published by SelectBooks, Inc.
For information address SelectBooks, Inc., New York, New York.

First Edition

ISBN 978-1-59079-490-6

Library of Congress Cataloging-in-Publication Data

Names: Brewer, Stephen C., 1952- author.
Title: What happened to moderation? : the Canyon Ranch common-sense guide to
  improving our health and treating illnesses in an age of extremes /
  Stephen C. Brewer, MD, ABFM, Medical Director, Canyon Ranch Wellness
  Resorts, Tucson, Arizona.
Description: New York : SelectBooks, [2019] | Includes bibliographical
  references and index.
Identifiers: LCCN 2018060836 | ISBN 9781590794906 (pbk. book : alk. paper)
Subjects: LCSH: Medicine, Popular. | Health.
Classification: LCC RC81 .B874 2019 | DDC 613--dc23 LC record available at
  https://lccn.loc.gov/2018060836

Book design by Janice Benight

Manufactured in the United States of America
10 9 8 7 6 5 4 3 2 1

I would like to dedicate this book to two very special women in my life: my older sister, Deborah, and my daughter, Elizabeth. Both of these women have been very instrumental in molding my life. Deborah helped guide me down my path to a medical career. Growing up I watched my father as a country veterinarian care for animals. At a young age this opened my eyes to the world of medicine. However, it was Deborah's continued excitement and passion for medicine as a practicing nurse that convinced me that medicine was the field I wanted to be in. Finally her strength and her character has always been a model to me as to who I wanted to aspire to be as an individual.

The other woman I would like to dedicate this book to, my daughter, Elizabeth, is emotionally one of the strongest individuals I have known. She has kept herself focused on being healthy all her life through exercise, diet, and avoiding all forms of negative habits and behaviors. She is one of the most positive people I know. She has shown me that the glass is always half full. I feel her greatest gift is her ability to see and treat all people the same no—matter what their race, gender orientation, or spiritual beliefs may be. She only sees the goodness in everyone's heart.

Contents

Foreword

Throughout my many years as a primary care physician, researcher, educator, and evidence-based practitioner, I have seen all forms of diets, health treatments, exercise regimens, and illness prevention strategies come and go. The answer to how and why these fads arise and then disappear is complicated and varied. In the answer to this question, however, lies one consistent theme—there's a lack of clear evidence to support or disclaim the benefits or harms of a new fad in health routines. In other words, there is significant uncertainty. When doubt exists, and something can be sold, many products for the latest trend in health improvement will enter the market. Complexity is introduced in order to differentiate a new fad from an old extreme that was "the latest rage."

The practice of evidence-based medicine (EBM) can be defined in its most simple form as physicians who practice medicine by making decisions based on evidence from well-designed and well-conducted research and who are aware when there is uncertainty about the benefits and harms of a treatment they offer to their patients. Unfortunately, it has been well established that much of what we recommend to patients throughout our field of health care is often not based on sound scientific studies. When the evidence based on research does not indicate a clear outcome, it becomes critical for a physician to summarize and communicate this information to patients to guide them to make decisions that are best for them. Obviously when we lack clear evidence, the interpretation and application of conclusions from medical research can be difficult.

In the world of wellness, with its focus on mindfulness, sleep, nutrition, exercise, and disease prevention, there is a growing body of scientific evidence to support or not support these various approaches to improving our health. The known evidence, however, is complex, and there can be tremendous gaps in the attainment of scientific proof to support the claims that are made. These gaps in our knowledge are often exploited by the market place by advocates of extreme or overly complex solutions to achieve wellness. These extreme ideas may sell well when more moderate and reasonable approaches seem boring and are less marketable. When was the last time we saw an exciting new sitcom about physicians showing patients how to eat balanced diets or demonstrating how patients can perform simple aerobic exercises like walking frequently? Not something likely to be the next HBO hit.

In my own personal life, as I attempt to stay healthy while working at a stressful job and raising a family, I have come to appreciate the importance of moderate and sustainable approaches. While the evidence for this is complex, when the information available is appropriately distilled down to its basics ingredients, it agrees with this message.

Maintaining a healthy routine then depends on a reality check of your life and your day-to-day constraints. Built into my regimen are what I call "bumps" along the way. A basic element of sustainability is planning for the inevitable occasions when I catch a cold or have a family emergency—the times we are unable to achieve our immediate wellness goals. This way, when we encounter some anticipated "bumps," we don't get discouraged and will continue on the path with our eyes on the long-term goal of wellness.

Over the years I have seen patients attempt aggressive therapies or complicated regimens to reduce weight, increase exercise capacity, or fight off newly developed medical conditions like pre-diabetes or mild hypertension. These extreme solutions are often not just unhelpful. They can actually be harmful. Patients often move on and off diets and exercise programs or adopt overly complicated solutions that are never sustainable. They then become upset and fall completely out of their routines.

Some of the main ingredients of achieving wellness are simplicity, moderation, and consistency. What Dr. Brewer has brilliantly done in writing his latest book, *What Happened to Moderation?*, is to efficiently review the base of scientific evidence behind the major fields of wellness to create a sensible guide to help all of us move toward a moderate path to improve and maintain good health. He nimbly tackles the basis for many examples of complex scientific evidence, including the gaps, to distill them into an understandable simple message. He then explores practical, sustainable, reasonable ways to achieve our goals. His approach is unique in a field where the more extreme solutions and "new" or complex ideas dominate the market. As a family-medicine physician with training in integrative medicine, and his vast experience working with patients at Canyon Ranch Wellness Resorts, Stephen blends various fields and offers clear steps to guide us.

The field of health care needs Dr. Brewer's ideas desperately. Whether it's overuse of technology, over-prescribing of medications, or new extreme exercise programs, we need to pause and ask serious questions regarding the benefits and harm of these treatments or regimens. Recent advances in medicine for such conditions as gastrointestinal reflux, physical pain, and depression have revolutionized how we care for patients and have improved the lives of millions of people. But when is too much medication prescribed or taken for too long? What are the true side effects and benefits of these new medications? When and how should we stop new therapies? These questions are just as important as the reasons to initiate a treatment. But we as a medical society have not dealt with this issue as well as we have with initiating a new treatment. Dr. Brewer has outlined the basic steps we can all take to reassess the indications, duration, and possible side effects of common treatments.

—THOMAS G. MCGINN, MD, MPH
SVP and Deputy Physician-in-Chief
Northwell Health
Executive Director, Office of the Provider Network
Professor and Chair of Medicine
Donald & Barbara Zucker School of Medicine at Hofstra/Northwell

Acknowledgments

I would like to acknowledge the following individuals who have inspired me and guided me down my path to completing this book. The first person I want to thank is my editor, Nancy Sugihara, who quickly understood the essence of this book and then spent tireless hours editing and adding to this book to make it the quality book it is today. I want to thank my publishers, Kenzi and Kenichi Sugihara, for believing in me to produce this book. I want to thank my book agent, Bill Gladstone, who helped me initiate this project. I want to thank the leadership at Canyon Ranch who have given me the support and space to be the best physician I can be. This includes Susan Docherty, CEO of Canyon Ranch, and Thomas Klein, President and COO of Canyon Ranch. I want to thank Gary Frost, PhD, for his support and guidance that he has given me from all his leadership roles at Canyon Ranch. I want to thank all the doctors and practitioners of Canyon Ranch both in Tucson and Lenox for their professionalism and their ability to continually educate me on the most current medical treatments and breakthroughs. I want to once again thank Mel and Enid Zuckerman for initially giving me the opportunity to work at Canyon Ranch. Finally I would like to thank all the kind workers at Starbucks who have been serving me coffee and chai lattes over the last two years as I sat in in their easy chairs writing this book.

Lifestyle Choices

Introduction

Today we are living in a world of extremes. Our politicians and electorate are either extreme right or extreme left. No one seems to want to compromise or find the middle ground. Television personalities are over the top with their loudness and brashness. Athletes feel they cannot just compete anymore. They have to win and win big. A person can't just be a good human. They have to be superhuman.

Unfortunately the field of health and wellness has not been different from the rest of the country. It too has embraced a path of extremism. For example, the public has been told by the "health experts" that the only food they eat should be vegetarian, gluten-free, dairy-free, and grown on an organic farm within two miles from their homes. They get the same kind of recommendations for exercising. A good routine is no longer going out for a two-mile run or lifting weights for thirty minutes. These days a person must take part in an exhaustive Spartan Run or a marathon for it to be considered an exercise. Workouts at CrossFit have become almost a religion. I have seen how this has created a big dilemma for many of my patients over the years who are on the fence about making healthy lifestyle changes. Many decide not to attempt to go down a path of improving their health because everything they have seen or heard points to extreme measures they must undertake to be healthy.

Pushing healthy behaviors to the extreme has the potential of developing health problems, not eliminating them. I have seen this with the overuse of food supplements and vitamins. Vitamin D is the classic example of this. The public has been told by the medical establishment to stay out of the sun because sun exposure is the number one cause of skin cancer. The general public has dutifully gone along with this recommendation. But instead of just decreasing their sun exposure, they try to avoid the sun altogether by carrying large umbrellas, slapping on thick coatings of SPF 60 suntan lotions, and covering up in blankets every time they go outside.

There can be severe consequences to going to this extreme of trying to eliminate all sun exposure. There is no natural food that has vitamin D in it. For our bodies to naturally obtain Vitamin D, we need to have the sun hit the skin and transform chemicals in the skin into vitamin D. Our bodies need Vitamin D because it is very important for bone health. Low levels of Vitamin D can be associated with osteoporosis, which is a loss of bone. If a person stays out of the sun, they are likely to be told they need to take a supplemental form of vitamin D. Unfortunately, many individuals will not take the appropriate replacement dosage. They will go to the extreme and take excessive amounts.

I'll always remember a patient's case presented to the medical students and residents when I was an intern during medical Grand Rounds. When the lights went down, the physician presenting the case projected an X-ray on the screen behind him. He then turned to face the medical staff in the auditorium and asked the question based solely on looking at this X-ray, "What did this person die of?" I had no idea, and none of my fellow staff members at the time had any idea either. The X-ray was of the chest and the abdomen that was peppered with white spots. It turned out those white spots were areas of calcium deposits. The lecturer told us that the person died of vitamin D toxicity from ingesting too much vitamin D. The excess vitamin D resulted in an elevated absorption of calcium from the gut. This eventually overwhelmed the person's organs and resulted in total organ failure. Yes, many of us need a supplemental vitamin D. However, we don't need to take an excess of vitamin D.

The practice of medicine has also been guilty of excesses and extremes. This can readily be seen with the overuse of pharmaceuticals. To start with, there has been an excess use of stimulants in the treatment of Attention Deficit Disorders. Up to one in five teenage boys is now diagnosed with this disorder. The majority of the boys and girls who are diagnosed with this problem are placed on medications. The number of prescriptions written to treat ADD in this country is staggering. These medications have the potential for causing a number of significant ill effects such as high blood pressure, cardiac arrhythmias, and the drugs prescribed have an especially high risk for abuse.

Depression in the past was commonly undertreated because of the unwanted side effects from the older antidepressant medications, such as fatigue and dry mouth. The newer antidepressants such as the SSRIs (Prozac is one) generally have a lower side-effect profile. Because of this, many individuals, even those with mild depression, were encouraged to start on these antidepressants. No one needed to feel even a little depressed when there were drugs that could treat it. After years of using these so-called "side effect-free medications," it has been found that these medications do have some unintended effects on the body. Some of the problems seen with the newer antidepressants are decreased libido and erectile dysfunction.

Another huge area of overuse of medication occurs with treatment of gastrointestinal disorders. We rarely visit our local pharmacy without needing to walk down a long aisle loaded with treatments for every gut issue known to modern medicine, including remedies for reflux disease, constipation, diarrhea, stomach acid, and gas. Before many of these drugs were made, many people suffered terribly with severe GI problems. These medical issues included serious maladies such as bleeding ulcers. Now, with so many of these remedies available over the counter, they are being overused. Immoderate use of these medications can result in problems like osteoporosis and abnormal gut bacteria.

Lastly, opiates have definitely been overprescribed. There are multiple reasons for the overuse of opiates, including the medications innate potential for abuse and the medical profession's overzealous treatment of pain. Our country is now in the midst of a severe opiate crisis. We are experiencing abuse at an exponential level. The potential side effects of using these medications is far worse than with most other drugs. This includes the potential for abuse and overdose, which has a high risk of death.

Over ten years ago I coauthored a book on Peak Performance called *The Everest Principle.* The core of the book was to improve a person's diet, their physical activity, and their emotional wellbeing to maximize their health. An example of this is interval training. With interval training people push themselves at intervals to their limit as long as they can. They will then slow down for a finite period of time and continue to repeat this process at intervals during their exercise program. By doing this form of exercise, an individual can maximize their fitness level. They will burn up twice as many calories as a regular cardiac workout and improve their overall fitness level. At that time I felt it was important to push oneself in order to excel in good health. But pushing yourself is one thing. Extending yourself beyond what is reasonable is something else.

After practicing medicine for over thirty-five years, I have witnessed in my own personal health and my patients' health that embracing a life of healthy living—including eating what we consider a good diet, doing regular exercise, and learning the best ways to cope with stress—can greatly improve our quality of life and decrease the risk of chronic diseases. I have also learned that the approach to our diet, exercise, and routines to conquer stress need to be one of moderation. Unfortunately, when we take aspects of our health practices to an extreme, there is often a negative consequence. And a moderate approach is not only more successful for improving our health. It is a much easier path to follow than an extreme regimen.

As a physician, I find that equally important as performing truly healthy habits is sustaining these habits. During my years of practicing medicine I have found that patients who approach their wellbeing from a point of view of moderation are much more likely to continue their healthy ways than those who go about their body improvement rituals at full throttle. People who push themselves to the extreme often have a difficult time maintaining their rigorous Spartan life and eventually revert back to their old unhealthy ways.

Engaging in a healthy lifestyle is a lifelong commitment, but it does not need to be an arduous endeavor. In this book I recommend a moderate approach to exercise and diet practices and to solving some common problems of illness. I look at extreme behaviors that have the potential for negative outcomes and offer alternative approaches. Hopefully you will be convinced to engage in reasonable and enjoyable routines and will consider my recommendations for dealing with some chronic health disorders.

1

Attainable Health and Fitness Goals

Isn't the sky the limit?

When making a decision to learn and commit to a healthier lifestyle, one should first look for attainable goals. As I discussed in my first book on peak performance, I feel it is important to push oneself in our goals to exercise for good physical conditioning and health. It should be something we work toward. However, to put forth goals that are exhausting and almost impossible to attain can consume our time to the point that it prevents us from doing those things we need to perform. It is okay to push your limits, but not to the point that it exhausts you.

One of the most extreme cases of this is the Quintuple Anvil Triathlon. This is five iron-man length races in five days. One iron man alone is a 2.4-mile swim, 112-mile bike ride and a marathon (26.22 miles). Are you kidding me?! A famous quote by Dr. Jay Lonsway appeared in the *New York Times* November 6, 2016, on page one of the Sports Section when he completed this insanely difficult race and said, "I know this is not good for my body, but it is good for my soul." I would say this is the ultimate extreme of competitive sports, but someone will come along and have an event that is even more insane. People, what are we doing? For years it was considered craziness to do an iron man, and now, what is next? All reason goes out the door with these kinds of extreme goals that have the potential to cause permanent health issues.

We hear stories of the death marches that prisoners took during the wars. One example is the Bataan Death March during WWII in which 60-80,000 POWs were marched by the Japanese to Balanga, resulting in the deaths of 2,500–10,000 Filipinos and 500–650 Americans. Certainly these excess exercise goals and programs are not death marches, but they do have the potential of having a negative impact on our bodies.

I must reiterate at this point that if you love to exercise long hours and find exhilaration in maintaining a life in such extremes, I am not here to talk you out of it.

I have a very good friend, William, who loves to compete in ironman competitions. He ranks high nationally in his age group. William loves it. To compete at this level he exercises at least two hours every morning and two hours every evening and at least seven hours on Saturdays. The major reason he is able to do this is that he has no children at home, and he has a very understanding wife. This becomes not just a hobby for him but another full-time job. For him this works, while for most of us this is totally unrealistic. This effort will place William in the upper 99 percentage of fitness and wellness. However, people performing one fifth of what he does, puts them in the top 95 percent of healthy individuals!

It is important for all of us to determine what the state of our health is and where we want it to be. If you look into the mirror, and after being brutally honest with yourself you are truly satisfied with the state of your health, then it is perfectly okay to declare that your goal is to maintain your present state of health. There is nothing wrong with this goal. It can be a great goal. The older we become, especially over the age of fifty, maintaining a healthy state can be a great accomplishment. However, if you are like most individuals who look in the mirror and don't especially like what you see, now is the time to make a change and focus on a higher goal of fitness.

But please don't start off with that "pie in the sky" thinking. When we do this, we often don't even attempt to really improve our health. Pick a small, easily attainable goal. For example, if you aren't exercising at all, just aim to get out and walk a mile four or five days a week. This is a great beginning. Once that is accomplished, then you can think about another attainable goal. That might be to decrease alcohol consumption to one drink a night instead of the usual two or three. After this, then the next goal could be to meditate three times a week for five minutes at a time. Now you will start to see the pattern. Each little goal can easily be attained and never seems insurmountable. If you keep up this pattern, in a few months you will often find yourself in a wonderful healthy space. I have been using this method successfully for years with my patients at Canyon Ranch.

I have also done this with my own personal health. I thought I was healthy when I first started working at Canyon Ranch. Then I compared myself to other people that worked at this phenomenal wellness resort. I realized that there were a lot of things I could do to make my health even better. I did not make those changes all at once. I slowly added healthy choices and eliminated bad health decisions. When I look back, I am shocked at how far I have come in my own goals of good health. If I had decided when I first started working at Canyon Ranch that I needed to make all these changes all at once, I most likely would never have started in the first place.

If you continue on this great path of wellness, you are likely to finally come to a point that you will need to stop pushing yourself and perhaps even need to back down some. A way to recognize that it is time for this is when what you are doing starts to become a grind and isn't fun anymore. I realized this personally when I was running four and a half miles every day during the week and eight to ten miles on the weekend. It was becoming a chore. I was so tired on Saturdays that I had to take long naps every Saturday afternoon to recover. Every time I ran I could not wait till I turned the last corner in front of my neighborhood because I knew I had less than one-half mile to complete my run. I dreaded getting up in the morning. I realized that the extra time it took to run that distance kept me from stopping at Starbucks on the way to work to grab a coffee, have an enjoyable conversation with the retired college professors from the University of Arizona, or do some writing. Also my old football injury that occurred in my leg was now acting up.

So I decided it was definitely time to back off from my routine. I decreased my weekly runs down to three miles and stopped the Saturday long run. If I did run on Saturday it was still just a three-mile run, even though I had time to run further. Suddenly my weekly runs were no longer a grind, and the Saturday run did not wipe me out for the rest of the day. I finally got back to going to the coffee house and having great intellectual conversations and not having the fatigue I experienced before. I was still exercising five days a week, doing a very healthy exercise program and my body loved it. I had a great goal for staying fit that I could maintain and enjoy without overdoing it.

A good example of a healthy obtainable goal is your goal for your body weight. Ideally your percent of body fat is a better means of determining a reasonable goal for what your body should be rather than what your actual weight is on the scales.

Despite knowing that a person's percentage of body fat is a better way of determining our state of health, our bathroom scales are still a good way to judge our overall health. If for years you have weighed 170 pounds but over the last one to two years you have gained a significant amount of weight and now you weigh 220 pounds, unless you decided to go to the weight room every day, and now look like you are ready to enter the Mr. Universe contest, odds are you have become quite unhealthy.

||||||||||||||||||||||||||||||||||||||||||||||||||||||||||||||||||||||||||||||||||||||||||||||||||||

ABOUT BODY WEIGHT

If you are blessed with a lot of muscle, you may weigh more than what a chart says is ideal but have low body fat, which is actually a lot healthier. If you have an accurate means of measuring body fat such as a dexa body composition or Bodpod, then the goal body fat for men is to be less than 25 percent and for women the goal is to be less than 38 percent body fat. The percentage of body fat measured on bathroom scales, electro-impedance devices, and calipers performed by fitness experts can grossly underestimate your actual body fat. At Canyon Ranch where I personally measure my patients with a dexa body composition machine, I get very surprised looks from my patients when I tell them what their actual percentage of body fat is.

||||||||||||||||||||||||||||||||||||||||||||||||||||||||||||||||||||||||||||||||||||||||||||||||||||

Now if you suddenly decide you want to get back to 170 pounds, that's a noble goal. However, after watching patients like this over the years, I've observed that they start off at full guns, and after a couple of weeks of working very hard on their diet and exercise, they weigh themselves and discover they have lost only two or three pounds. At that point they realize their goal is still 48 pounds away, and they often give up right there and then. By initially making the goal to be to 200 pounds, a person doesn't feel discouraged as easily if they aren't making the rapid progress they were hoping for. They won't give up. As soon as the 200-pound barrier is broken, it's then time for the 190-pound barrier to be broken. If they make it to 190 and they can't seem to move any further, I like point out to these patients that at 190 pounds they are so much healthier than they were at 220. The result is often that instead of stopping their healthy lifestyle, they maintain it. And many times, to their surprise, they will very slowly continue to lose weight.

There are always dynamic changes that present themselves, and these can make your goals much more difficult to attain. Suddenly you might have a sick parent that you must care for. Or your child needs to be taken daily to a new job. Perhaps you have also been given a huge new project at work. All these things can interfere with your exercise routines. Since these are all "normal" life happenings, we need to not be discouraged when they occur. This is actually what the real normal is. When everything is running smoothly this is not the norm. So be prepared for bumps because they will happen and be sure to put those "bumps" into your equation when you are trying to determine your goals. This way the knowledge that these bumps will occur will not cause you to become too discouraged on your path to accomplish your goals.

Finally, if your goals are always easy to attain, and you really never feel you are pushing yourself, maybe it's time to step it up a notch. Remember that the body likes to be pushed a little so that it can respond and build itself up to be stronger. No one increases their muscle mass by lifting the same amount of weight each time they exercise. The body needs to break things down so we can build it up to be stronger. This all comes back again to pursuing good health through an approach of moderation. Push and bend—don't break.

THE MODERATION APPROACH TO ATTAINABLE GOALS

1. Don't make goals for improving your health that are unattainable.

2. Be sure to set your goals to push yourself at least a little.

3. To improve your health, it may be much easier and more satisfying to make small incremental goals rather than choosing huge, difficult, and likely unrealistic goals. This will give you a more positive outlook since it will prevent you from becoming disappointed and then reversing everything you have already accomplished.

4. When you have goals to be more healthy but realize achieving them is much more arduous than you originally thought, don't stop altogether. Just back down a little with your choice of goals and continue on.

5. Remember that maintaining your present health goals as you age can be a great goal.

2

Exercising

Which routines are best for my health?

Regular, moderate aerobic exercise has been shown to be one of the best means to prevent chronic disease that we know of. Moderate exercise is defined as working out approximately one hundred fifty minutes a week (thirty minutes five days a week) at an intensity that a person can get their heart rate up to 70 to 85 percent of their predicted maximum heart rate (the number of 220 minus your age is the predicted maximum heart rate). There is no pharmaceutical drug that has the overall impact in the prevention of disease that regular exercise can give. It is one of the few things that has been shown to lower the risk for dementia. It decreases a person's risk for cancer by 50 percent. It decreases a person's risk for developing coronary artery heart disease by helping to lower blood pressure, decreasing cholesterol, lowering inflammation in the body, and decreasing the risk for blood clotting.

Unfortunately, there is a misconception by many people that exercising one hundred fifty minutes a week is not enough. There are many people who believe a person must exercise at least one hundred fifty minutes every day, and if they aren't working out at least that much, they aren't really exercising. That same group of individuals will ridicule others who are only running 5Ks instead of one half or full marathons. I personally have run for most of my adult life. One of my biggest pet peeves over the years has been that whenever I have an initial conversation with a fellow runner, invariably one of the first things they ask me is: "How many marathons have you run?" Well, I have never run a marathon, and I never intend to run one. If you are someone who has run a marathon I applaud you. It is one of the most demanding events in sports. However, just because I haven't run a marathon certainly does not mean I am not a runner. Whenever I am asked that question of how many marathons I have run, I often remind them that the very first marathoner, who ran the 26-plus miles after the battle of Marathon, to announce victory of the Greeks over the Persians to the king, collapsed and died from the run!

In the world of exercise, more is often assumed to be better. Unfortunately, events such as marathons, ultramarathons, iron-man distance triathlons, and very long distance bicycle races can result in a lot of health issues. The most common ailments that occur with excess exercise are musculoskeletal injuries. These injuries can be anything from muscle strains to stress fractures. They are called "stress" fractures (fracture is a doctor's language for a broken bone) because the repetitive pounding that endurance athletes place on their bones can result in cracks in their bones.

Over the years I have volunteered as a team physician in high school sports. Because of this involvement, a lot of amateur athletes have gravitated to me as patients. It was not unusual for me to see patients who were in their last weeks of training for a marathon and complaining of leg pain. It usually occurred when they were increasing the mileage of their runs when preparing for the long distance of the marathon. That extra wear and tear on their bones often resulted in stress fractures. When that happens all those months of training were all for naught because they had to stop running until the fracture healed.

I had one running partner who had been increasing his running distance for an upcoming marathon, and he developed leg pain. He would not tell anybody about the pain and continued to run. The excessive running caused a hairline fracture of his large, lower leg bone called his tibia. He proceeded to run the marathon, and his hairline stress fracture shattered during the race. Instead of a hairline fracture of bone that just needed to be in a cast and immobilized, he now had a fracture that was a compound fracture (a compound fracture is when a break is so severe that the bone breaks through the skin) and required surgery with a metal rod placement. Because of this he had to quit running for two years.

A recent finding is the potential for cardiac disease in individuals taking part in endurance training. This has really shocked the endurance world. The last thing that endurance athletes thought they would have to worry about was their hearts. Isn't exercise good for your heart? Well, exercise in moderation absolutely is good for your heart, but when the heart is exposed to the rigors of endurance training there is a potential negative outcome. In endurance training the heart is exposed to a much higher volume of blood return than normal. This can overload the right side of the heart (where venous blood returns to the heart) and result in injury. The heart usually recovers in a week. However, it has been shown that recurrent volume overload can cause scarring of the heart. This scaring can ultimately cause the heart muscle to dysfunction and may decrease the ability of the heart to pump. This may be severe enough that the heart can decompensate and result in heart failure. This has also been associated with cardiac rhythm disturbances and coronary artery disease.[1]

It has been known that exercise has been associated with increased testosterone and increased libido.[2] Being in great shape has therefore been a means to improve one's love life. Going for a run and then coming home and having sexual bliss is a great and wonderful thing. Over the years one of the first great benefits my patients have told me about their newfound exercise program is that they now have an improved sex life.

So what about endurance athletes when it comes to testosterone and libido? If a little is good, wouldn't a lot be even better? It looks like the opposite is happening. Studies have shown that endurance training can actually decrease testosterone production.[3] And with a decrease in testosterone there is the potential for a lowered libido. An article written in the journal of *Medicine and Science in Sports and Exercise* presents a study showing that exposure to higher levels of chronic, intense, and greater durations of endurance training on a regular basis is associated with a decreased libido score in men. In this study a group of 1,100 men, who did not have ED, were involved with endurance running and cycling. Those men that engaged in the highest intensity training had the lowest libido scoring compared to the group of men participating in the lowest and midrange intensity training who had the highest libido scoring.[4]

When young women perform excessive exercise, it is not unusual to develop amenorrhea. Amenorrhea is defined as not having a menstrual flow for one or more menstrual periods. When amenorrhea occurs because of excessive exercise it is called exercise associated amenorrhea (EAA). These are women who have exercised a great deal and often restrict their diet at the same time. This then can result in extreme weight loss. It is the most common cause of secondary amenorrhea in female athletes. This condition has been found to effect 5 to 25 percent of female athletes (some studies have said it to be as high as 44 percent). The pathophysiology of this problem is related to the production of the of the hormone, GnRH (gonadal releasing hormone). This hormone is produced in the area of the brain called the hypothalamus. Its job is to signal the pituitary gland to secrete two hormones called LH (luteinizing hormone) and FSH (follicle stimulating hormone). These hormones affect the ovaries to mature the eggs and release them as well as in the production of estrogen and progesterone. GnRH is released from the hypothalamus in pulsations every sixty to ninety minutes. With vigorous exercise and restrictive dieting the hormone is released less frequently and in not the same pulsations. Therefore it does not effectively stimulate the ovarian follicles to ovulate and produce hormones. The resultant is the lack of a menstrual period.

One of the bigger problems that can occur with the decreased production of hormones is seen in bone health. Estrogen is involved in maintaining healthy bones. Lack of estrogen can cause bone loss, which increases the risk of bone fracture. This has become such a big problem that the combination of amenorrhea, osteoporosis, and disordered eating has been given the name of "The Female Athlete Triad."

Heat injuries are another consequence of extreme athletic behavior. They occur because the athlete does not supply the body the proper fluids and nourishment it may need during excessive exercise. There are three basic heat injuries that can occur with excess exercise. They are: heat exhaustion, heat injury, and heat stroke.

- **Heat exhaustion**—Heat exhaustion is characterized by the inability to maintain adequate cardiac output (volume of blood pumped by the heart) due to strenuous physical exercise and environmental heat stress. Acute dehydration may be present, but it is not required for the diagnosis.

- **Heat injury**—Heat injury is defined as an exertional heat illness with evidence of both hyperthermia and end organ damage, but without any significant neurologic manifestations. The absence of neurologic findings distinguishes the diagnosis from heat stroke,

- **Heat stroke**—Heat stroke is a multisystem illness characterized by central nervous system (brain and spinal cord) dysfunction and additional organ and tissue damage (Examples include acute kidney injury, liver injury, muscle breakdown) in association with high body temperatures.

Causes of these heat related injuries are as follows:

- Strenuous exercise in high temperature and humidity
- Lack of acclimatization
- Poor physical fitness
- Obesity
- Dehydration
- Medications (which includes anticholinergic agents, antiepileptic agents, antihistamines, decongestants, phenothiazines, tricyclic antidepressants, amphetamines, and ergogenic stimulants like ephedrine, lithium, diuretics, beta blockers, and ethanol)

Another major concern about excess exercise is a rare muscle breakdown disease called rhabdomyolysis. This usually occurs with individuals who have been deconditioned and suddenly do an excessive workout. It does not necessarily occur after long runs but has been observed after a strenuous spinning class. It has been seen most commonly with deconditioned soldiers going through boot camp. It is now more common in the general public because of the big push toward extreme exercise like the Spartan runs, etc. Our muscles need time to adjust to higher intensity exercise programs.

Rhabdomyolysis is the breakdown of muscle tissue and the release of muscle breakdown products into the bloodstream. A person's creatinine kinase blood levels will become extremely elevated. This is an enzyme found in muscle tissue. The kidneys can be affected by this sudden pouring of this enzyme into the bloodstream. These enzymes need to be filtered by the kidney. Usually the kidneys can handle the creatinine that is produced from normal aging and breakdown of muscle tissue. However, in those incidents in which such a large load goes to the kidneys, they can be overwhelmed, and kidney failure can occur. The muscles most commonly associated with this syndrome are the proximal muscles that are the ones closest to the trunk, such as the shoulder and thighs muscles. The classic triad for this injury is severe muscle pain, weakness, and dark urine. If this triad is found, one needs to seek medical attention immediately.

So if excess exercise is bad, what is good exercise? Exercise in moderation! This magical word can be the key to a healthy and enjoyable life. This is what I have practiced myself personally for the majority of my whole adult life. It is also the philosophy and recommendation I have given to my patients over the last thirty-five years of practicing medicine. I exercise in moderation by going out for a three-mile run on relatively flat surfaces five days a week. That takes me about thirty minutes. I am not breaking any land speed records, but this is not why I do it. I don't record my time each time I run, since I am just happy to know that I was able to still run the distance. Until a year ago I was running four to five miles at a times and realized I was excessively tired for the rest of the day, and I had significant muscle and joint pain. When I decreased my distance to three miles, suddenly my post exercise achiness and fatigue disappeared.

Everyone needs to find that happy medium where they are pushing themselves for at least twenty-five to thirty minutes but do not have any lingering post exercise fatigue or muscle and joint pain. I also lift weights two days a week for thirty minutes. With this shortened time I don't have to get up as early, and therefore my exercising doesn't cut into my sleep time. (We will discuss later the importance of getting adequate sleep in maintaining good health.) If you have time restraints when you exercise, you can maximize this time by doing interval training. Interval training is certainly not a must in order to be healthy, but it can help increase your fitness level, which is important for easier weight loss if that is an issue or goal for you.

Many people who may be on the fence about exercising to improve their health are often turned off when they hear individuals talk about exercising only in terms of Spartan runs, marathons, and CrossFit. I have seen this response over and over again with my patients who look at these extremes in lifestyle and decide it's just not worth the effort to be healthy. They will hear people talk about exercise in terms of hours not minutes. My patients have heard over-the-top, beating of the chest statements from people at work in discussions over a morning coffee about one-hundred-mile bike rides and multiple marathons. People listening to this chatter often feel exercising would be way too difficult and time-consuming to do, let alone maintain these routines over time. Once again, look to an ideal of moderation as your guide. Exercising thirty minutes a day, five days a week at a good intensity will give incredible benefits without compromising a person's time or expending excess energy.

So what ultimately happens when so many people hear about these arduous exercise programs? They often do nothing. I have to sit and explain and re-educate my patients all the time that exercise, even for fifteen minutes, can have a huge effect on improving their health. I want to make a point here that I am not against endurance exercise, and I don't want to discourage you from running marathons or going to CrossFit. If you love doing it, and you are able to do it without injuring yourself, please proceed. I know of one individual who loves CrossFit so much that whenever he goes out of town he always locates one and goes to the local Crossfit facility to work out so he does not interrupt his exercise routine. It has given him a sense of community, and he loves the strenuous exercise. What I am trying to emphasize is that a person can be very healthy and decrease their risk of disease without pursuing intense exercise routines.

So, in summary, if excess exercise has potential negative consequences what is effective, maintainable alternative? It's moderate exercise! This can be the key to a healthy, enjoyable life.

HEALTHY, MODERATE APPROACHES TO EXERCISE INCLUDE THE FOLLOWING:

1. Perform cardiovascular exercise a minimum of three days a week. I prefer five days, but will settle for three if a person's life is so busy they just don't have the time for this. Types of cardiovascular exercises are running, biking, swimming, and working on an elliptical, treadmill, or stationary bike. In order for these exercises to be a cardiovascular exercise, they need to be performed at an intensity in which you increase your heart rate between 70 and 85 percent of its predicted maximum rate (subtract your age from 220 to get your maximum heart rate). This exercise needs to be thirty minutes or more. Exercising longer than an hour starts to increase your risk of injury or disease.

2. You can increase the effects of your exercise if you increase the intensity of the exercise at intervals during the exercise. The simple version of this is to increase the intensity of your exercise program to above 85 percent of your predicted maximum heart rate (220 minus your age). The best way to determine you have hit this threshold is that you will notice that your breathing rate will suddenly increase. Try to stay at this level as long as you can, for approximately sixty seconds, and then slow back down to the cardio pace of 70 to 85 percent of your predicted maximum heart rate. Maintain this for a few minutes, and then repeat this pattern over and over

for twenty to thirty minutes. By performing this type of exercise you will have the ability to burn up more calories and increase your fitness level. This type of exercise program allows you to exercise for a shorter period of time. The author's note here is that as I get older and am now in my 60s, I rarely perform this type of workout because with the higher intensity there is a higher risk of muscle strain.

3. Perform some type of weight-training program two days a week. This is more important to us as we get older because of the increased loss of skeletal muscle mass. Please do not replace a cardio day with a weight-training day. You must keep three days sacred with cardio exercise for disease prevention. If you are doing weight training for the first time, please be trained by a certified trainer. Otherwise you could get hurt. Be sure to focus on the large muscle groups such as chest, back and legs. These burn up the most calories. If you have time it is certainly fine to work on the smaller muscle groups.

3

Dietary Decisions

Should I follow a strict diet to improve my health?

Restrictive dieting, like excesses in exercise, can cause significant ill effects. A classic negative effect of restrictive dieting was seen when Ashton Kutcher tried getting into character as Steve Jobs in the movie, "Jobs." He tried to emulate Steve Jobs by placing himself on the same diet Steve Jobs often placed himself on. This was a purely all fruit diet. A few days before filming was to start, Ashton developed severe abdominal pain and was rushed to the hospital. He was found to have pancreatitis. Eating mostly or only fruit can cause deficiencies in essential vitamins and nutrients, including calcium, iron, zinc, and vitamins D, B12, and other B vitamins. It can also be very low in protein and fatty acids.

Vegetarian Diets

These popular restrictive diets vary according to the degree of avoidance of foods of animal origin. A strict vegetarian diet consists of cereals, legumes, vegetables, fruits, and nuts. This diet excludes dairy products, animal meats, and eggs. Other kinds of limited vegetarian diets include the following:

1. **Semi-vegetarian:** Meat is occasionally used.

2. **Lacto-ovo-vegetarian:** Eggs, milk, and milk products are included. (lacto = dairy; ovo = eggs)

3. **Lacto-vegetarian:** Milk and milk products are included, but no eggs or meat are eaten.

4. **Vegan:** All animal products, milk products, and eggs are excluded. Some vegans refrain from honey and will not use leather or wool products.

I am always amazed at the latest fads in diets. Humans are very funny animals. They always want to be the first on the block to try out the newest "thing," and that certainly includes the newest diet craze. Humans often feel if something is new it must be better. Many of these diets are extreme and very restrictive. Each one seems more extreme than the next. There is one major word of caution when it comes to restrictive dieting, and that is to be careful with these diets when it comes to children. As a family physician I have seen parents go on these restrictive diets, and they think that because a particular restrictive diet is supposed to be good for them, it must be good for their children. Poorly planned or severely restricted diets can lead to nutrient deficiencies that may compromise or delay growth in children.[5, 6]

The other concern is if you start a child on restrictive dieting you may be opening the door to abnormal eating patterns, like bulimia or anorexia. Therefore, if you are a parent, before you consider placing your child on a restrictive diet, please check with the child's pediatrician or family physician to be sure it is okay for your child to be on it.

What does it mean to eat moderately and well? To begin with, we certainly don't need to overeat. Unless we are bears getting ready to hibernate, there are little advantages to overeating. It often leads to being overweight, which increases your risk for multiple chronic disease states such as diabetes and heart disease. We already talked about the negatives of a restrictive diet, but what is a good, well-rounded, "moderate" diet?

A Healthy Diet Is What I Term "Eating in Moderation"

There are some very simple rules to healthy eating in moderation.

Rule #1: Eat a colorful meal. What do I mean by that? It means eating colorful fruits and vegetables. If you look down at your plate and it looks like a black and white movie, that is your first clue that it is unhealthy. It should look like a bouquet of colorful flowers. There should be beautiful greens (containing folic acid and iron), bright reds from tomatoes (good sources of lycopene) and red peppers (high in vitamin C and other vitamins and minerals, and orange colors from carrots (rich in beta-carotene for our body to make vitamin A). And this can accompany a bowl of red, blue, and purple berries (great antioxidants!).

Rule #2: Learn About the Different Types of Protein. A huge fallacy is that you can't get protein without it being real meat. One can get protein from such non-meats as mushrooms, soy, and nuts. If you are not a vegetarian and you decide you want to eat meat, one of your first choices should be fish. It is a good protein with healthy fat content. Yes, there is a concern about mercury, but if go to the Monterey Aquarium website it will direct you to those fish that contain the least amount of mercury. Typically avoid predatory fish like shark, tuna, and swordfish. This could then be followed by chicken or turkey. Try to avoid red meat. It doesn't mean you can't occasionally have a piece of lean red meat. I feel once a week is plenty. There are too many negatives associated with red meat, which includes increasing our cholesterol level. The most recent negative associated with red meat is the chemical called TMAO (Trimethylamine N-oxide) that is produced by red meat in the gut and that can lead to heart disease.[7]

Rule #3: Learn portion control. This is another major aspect of moderate, healthy eating. Serving sizes should be no larger than your fist. A simple test to help you determine if the amount you are eating is appropriate is to test yourself when you are getting close to finishing your meal. If you feel stuffed, it is a no-brainer—you have served yourself too much food. If you feel you are full, you also have eaten too much. It takes about fifteen to twenty minutes for the brain to recognize how full we really are. The key is to stop eating when you feel you really could eat another serving, but know you'll be glad if you don't.

Rule #4: Do your best to eat breakfast. This is a simple logical step. Breakfast gives you fuel for the day. It is not the end of the world if you don't eat breakfast, but I don't advise it. If you don't eat breakfast, then at least try to have a healthy mid-morning snack. A simple snack would be a fruit with a protein such as nuts or soy.

Rule #5: Do not eat a huge meal at the end of the day. And this last meal should not be late in the day (after 7:30 or 8:00). This is very logical, also. If you eat a large meal at the end of the day, you aren't going to need those calories to fuel you for any activities. Those calories won't be burned up, and the body will potentially store this as excess fat.

Rule #6: Eat your fruits and vegetables. Duh! Momma was right on this one. It is relatively easy to eat fruit with all your meals, but eating vegetables for breakfast from an American breakfast seems hard to swallow. The reality is that other cultures eat vegetables with their first meal of the day. I remember getting up and having breakfast when I was spending time in Turkey and seeing all the vegetables that were sitting out on the buffet table. I have to admit it took me a couple days to get used to it, but by the third day I was actually eating vegetables for breakfast. The general rule is to have at least five servings of fruits and vegetables a day. That isn't as hard as it sounds. Just be sure to eat every meal with one or two servings of fruits and vegetables.

Rule #7: Limit your starches and breads. That means eating less potatoes (especially white potatoes) and breads.

The Origin of Recommending Four Food Groups in Our Daily Diet

When I was growing up, one of my first jobs in life was to get up in the morning and to go to the front door and bring in the milk that the milkman had delivered earlier in the morning. It was always sitting there outside the front door in clear-glass quart bottles. The milkman had stopped by our house about 5:00 a.m., picked up the empty milk bottles my mom set out the night before, and delivered the fresh bottles of milk. Everyone drank milk. Every meal would be served with a glass of milk, and we were often given a glass of milk at bedtime to help us fall asleep. All the kids had a minimum of three glasses of milk a day. It seemed like every day during mealtime my mom would tell me that I had to drink my milk to build up my bones. Otherwise my bones were going to fall apart.

In school in our science class we talked about the four food groups, of which dairy was one of them. I came from a rural area where my father was a country veterinarian who treated dairy cattle all the time. It seemed perfectly natural that milk should be one of the four major food groups. Little did I know at the time that it was only a food group because the American Dairy Association had a huge lobby in Washington.

The basic food groups were transformed over the years by the US Department of Agriculture. The first USDA food guide presented in 1916 written by a nutritionist emphasized vitamins and minerals. The guide was revised over the years to help families during wartime food rationing and was also revised in 1941 when the National Academy of Science devised RDA (Recommended Dietary Allowances). There was a lot of confusing contradictory advice issued in the food guides, so the multiple food groups were revised by the US Dept of Agriculture in 1956 to recommend the basic four food groups, which we base our diets on:

1. Milk
2. Meat
3. Fruit & Vegetables
4. Grains

In the 1970s research showed there was an increased risk for chronic diseases such as heart disease and diabetes from diets high in fats and sodium. Because of this, the "Food Pyramid" was developed. It took a long time to make this dietary model. It was originally introduced in 1988, but since there was so much pushback by the meat and dairy producers, it wasn't until 1992 that it was finally brought to the general public.[8]

It promoted the consumption of complex carbohydrates and discouraged all fats and oils. It soon became evident that the pyramid was flawed because it did not distinguish different kinds of fats, and some are the monosaturated and certain polyunsaturated fats, which are healthy and reduce cholesterol rather than increasing it[9] and saturated fats that can increase the risk of cardiovascular disease.[10]

Dairy vs. Nondairy

To understand the pros and cons of milk, it is first important to know the actual content of milk. Typical raw milk has the following average composition:

- 3.20 percent protein

- 3.65 percent fat
- 4.75 percent lactose (milk sugar)
- 0.65 percent minerals (calcium, etc.)
- 87.75 percent water

The amount of fat varies from one milk product to another. Skim milk, called fat-free, can have no more than .2 percent fat, and there is low-fat milk with 1 percent fat, reduced-fat milk that contains 2 percent fat, and whole milk that is milk with 3.65 percent fat. The type of fat is approximately 65 percent saturated, 30 percent monounsaturated, and 5 percent polyunsaturated fatty acids. Next is the milk sugar, which is lactose. Lactose is a disaccharide sugar which is made up of two sugars: glucose and galactose. These sugars are held together by a single bond. The last major component of milk is the protein. It contains two proteins, casein (80 percent) and whey (20 percent).

Since nutritionists and consumers frequently talk about "dairy or nondairy" products, the first thing we should address is the milk allergy commonly observed when eating cow dairy produce. What a lot of people think is milk allergy is actually lactose intolerance and not a true food allergy. People often say they can't tolerate dairy because they are "allergic" to it. This may mean one of two things. They may have a true food allergy to the milk protein or they are not able to break down the milk sugar so it can be absorbed into the body. Actual cow's milk allergy is the most common food allergy in children. It is not as common in adults. Even though it is the most common true food allergy it is still seen in only about 2 percent of infants. Food allergy presents with a wide range of clinical syndromes due to immunologic responses to cow's milk proteins. The symptoms associated with cow's milk allergy are varied. About 50 to 70 percent have cutaneous (skin) symptoms, 50 to 60 percent gastrointestinal symptoms, and about 20 to 30 percent respiratory symptoms.[11,12]

The most common reason people can't tolerant dairy products is not because they have an allergic reaction. It's because they can't digest the milk sugar, lactose. As I said earlier, milk sugar is a disaccharide, which is a combination of two simple sugars: glucose and galactose. The bond that holds those two sugars together must be broken first before those sugars can be absorbed across the gut. The enzyme that breaks the bond is called lactase. Once the bond is broken, the two simple sugars can then be absorbed into the body across the gut. If a person does not make enough of the enzyme, lactase, then the lactose stays in the gut and the bacteria in the gut use it for food, and this produces a lot of gas and bloating. That is not an allergic reaction. It is a result of the body's inability to digest the milk sugar. With an allergic reaction any amount of milk can cause a reaction to the protein.

With lactose intolerance a person may be able to take some milk but not a lot of milk (one scoop of ice cream versus two scoops). It all depends on how much of the enzyme, lactase, a person makes. There is a relative lactose intolerance when a person, especially children, has a viral gastroenteritis with a lot of diarrhea. The lactase enzyme is swept away with the diarrhea. It takes a few days after a virus resolves for a person to rebuild his or her lactase stores. That is why I always have my patients avoid milk products for at least two days following the resolution of a diarrhea.

So outside of lactose intolerance and true milk allergy is there any reason to avoid dairy? Yes, certainly if a person is trying to lose weight, it is important to limit the dairy product, cheese. As you will shortly read in this chapter, cheese is packed with calories.

A MODERATION APPROACH TO EATING DAIRY PRODUCTS

1. If you are truly allergic to dairy protein, you must avoid dairy altogether. Remember that even minimal amounts of dairy protein can cause a reaction.

2. If you are lactose intolerant, certainly taking the enzyme lactase with any dairy product can significantly decrease the gastrointestinal symptoms of bloating and gassiness. There is a limit on how much the lactase enzyme will work, so one scoop of ice cream may be okay, but a whole bowl of ice cream can still be deadly. Lactase can be found over the counter at any pharmacy.

3. Milk fat is 60 percent saturated fat, which has long been known as a risk factor for causing heart disease. Therefore whole milk with every meal, which is what I use to drink, is a no-no. One serving of dairy a day seems to cause little, if any, problems.

4. Limit cheeses. They have high calorie and salt content.

Weight-Loss Diets: The Low Fat vs. Low Carbs Debate

Let's look at weight-loss diets in terms of moderation. The number of weight-loss diets seems to be limitless. You are told that every one of these diets is going to help you lose weight and keep you healthy into your 90s. I used to be amazed at the number of times my patients would attribute a dramatic weight loss to some brand-new diet that some movie star was promoting. How could so many diets be successful but the obesity epidemic remain exponential? The answer is often quite simple. From the words of my wise old Integrative medicine professor, Dr. Andrew Weil, almost anyone that places themselves on a basic structured diet that they are able to stick to, and not waiver from for a considerable time, will more often than not be able to lose quite a bit of weight. But if we don't follow a diet structure, we humans have the tendency to pursue a graze-diet and eat whatever is within our arm's reach.

One of the biggest areas of extremes in diets has been the divide of the low-fat vs. low-carb diets. This has been an ongoing debate in nutrition for years. Even before I started to work at Canyon Ranch this debate was ongoing. In the late 40s and 50s when heart disease started to increase and autopsies showed significant amounts of cholesterol-laden plaque in the arteries, the big culprit was felt to be fat. With this information there was a push to decrease the fat content in our foods. That is when butter was replaced by margarine. Little did we know that in our haste to eliminate the dreaded butter, we created a new monster, trans fats, which may be even more atherogenic (causing formation of fatty plaques known as "hardening" of the arteries) than the saturated fats.

Later in 1972 along comes the famous Dr. Atkins' book, *Dr. Atkins' Diet Revolution,* which states that fat is no longer the problem. It is those dreaded carbohydrates that are causing all the ills in our bodies. By simply decreasing those potentially harmful carbs, we would lose weight and become healthy. Here we went again from one extreme to another.

Let's look at both of their arguments. Then in the end, we can see where the moderation approach is really the best approach to being healthy and having healthy weight.

Low-Fat Diets

Why is a low-fat diet considered an important recommendation by many cardiologists and nutritionists? It doesn't take a rocket scientist for someone to equate the excess fatty deposits found inside the arteries of a people with cardiovascular disease, such as heart attacks and strokes, with excess fat intake.[13] Scientific studies dating from the late 1940s showed a correlation between high-fat diets and high-cholesterol levels, suggesting that a low-fat diet might prevent heart disease in high-risk patients.

The beginnings of the popularity of low-fat diets began in the 1920s when women in society were coming out of the Victorian Age of high collars and long dresses into fashions of more revealing clothing. Many women were interested in improving their bodies that were now exposed to everyone. The general public took it upon themselves to find ways to change their eating habits. Regular columns in the newspapers featured diets that could improve their appearance. Even back then they were counting calories. The educated public knew that fat was 9 calories per gram and sugar was 4 calories per gram.[14]

The Origins of "The Mediterranean Diet"

The first major focus on fat and health came from the *Seven Country Study* done by Ancel Keys. In 1947 Ancel Keys started his work on this outcome study because at that time seemingly healthy middle-aged male executives were dropping dead from heart attacks on the streets of America. He wanted to know what the difference was between those who had heart attacks and those that stayed well.[15]

In 1951 Keys was on a sabbatical in Italy where he did a study of Neapolitan workers because he was told they rarely had heart attacks. He studied laborers and executives to analyze their blood and diet. Keys found that the laborers who had lower levels of cholesterol than the executives had a much lower risk of developing heart attacks. He then looked at seven countries and found a pattern of lower levels of heart attacks in the countries around the Mediterranean, Japan, and natives of South Africa.[16]

A formal study was started in 1958 to study these factors in the seven countries. The main hypothesis was that the rate of coronary disease in populations and individuals would vary in relation to their physical characteristics and lifestyle, particularly in fat composition of their diet in relation to their to serum cholesterol, or the total blood cholesterol levels. The results of the study showed that high levels of cholesterol, high blood pressure, diabetes, and smoking are universal risk factors for coronary heart disease.[17]

During the study it was recognized that the eating pattern that was commonly seen in Italy and Greece in the 1950s and '60s, which is now popularly called "The Mediterranean Diet," was associated with low rates of coronary heart disease and all-cause mortality (the number of deaths in a population from all causes during a specified period). The studies of the elderly also showed that a healthy diet and lifestyle (sufficient physical activity, no smoking, and moderate alcohol consumption) was associated with a low risk of cardiovascular disease and all-cause mortality. For the elderly, a healthy diet and sufficient physical exercise may also postpone cognitive decline and decrease the risk of depression.

With a Mediterranean diet the fat content was significantly less, but more importantly the fat consumed was rarely from animal fat. The fat came mostly from olive oil, avocados, and nuts. This was a very palatable diet.

Going Even Further with Very Strict Rules for a Low-Fat Diet

Of course with our Western habits of immoderate thinking, this did not go far enough. Americans had to take an extreme view of the value of low fat. All fat became evil.

One of the exaggerated interpretations of the findings about healthy eating came from Dr. Caldwell Esselstyn of the highly respected Cleveland Clinic. In his 2007 book *Preventing and Reversing Heart Disease* he lists the following very strict rules:

- You may not eat anything that has a mother or a face (no meat, poultry, or fish).
- You cannot eat dairy products.
- You must not consume oil of any kind.
- Generally you cannot eat nuts or avocados.

||||||||||||||||||||||||||||||||||||||||||||||||||||||||||||||||||||||||||||||||||||||||||||||||||||||||||||||||||||||||||||||||||

ANCEL KEYS

Ancel Keys (January 26, 1904 – November 20, 2004) was an American physiologist who studied the influence of diet on health lived to the age of 100. He was the founder of K rations distributed to the soldiers during WW II. After the war he organized and was the lead researcher in the now famous Seven Country Study of the diets and health of 12,000 healthy middle-aged men from many countries to discover the reasons for arterial blockages that cause heart attacks.* He was essentially the originator of the Mediterranean diet. He received two PhDs; his first was in oceanography and biology from UC Berkeley and his second in physiology from Cambridge University. He was credited for founding in 1939 what became a world-famous research facility, the Laboratory of Physiological Hygiene at the University of Minnesota School of Public Health, and he was its director for 33 years.**

||||||||||||||||||||||||||||||||||||||||||||||||||||||||||||||||||||||||||||||||||||||||||||||||||||||||||||||||||||||||||||||||||

---

* https://en.wikipedia.org/wiki/Ancel_Keys#Early_physiology_studies

** Jane Brody, "Dr. Ancel Keys, 100, Promoter of Mediterranean Diet. Dies," *New York Times*, November 23, 2004.

The typical Mediterranean diet has about 30 percent fats. Esselstyn's diet proposes a fat content that is less than 15 percent. This is a significant reduction in fat. One's taste of foods is radically changed by this. Most humans are very much hardwired for fat consumption. This is likely related to the fact that fat is 9 calories per gram vs. 4 calories per gram for carbs. Those cave people that went for the fat were given way more calories to survive. When we eat food with virtually no fat, it is often tasteless and very hard to eat.

However, in spite of the skepticism of many medical professionals about the wisdom of this strict vegan diet, as a physician I will still recommend this diet for those individuals who have progressive atherosclerosis despite having traditional medical or surgical treatments and following a healthy diet. This is not a preventative diet for those individuals. It becomes a therapeutic diet. It is in fact a survival diet, and in many cases I have seen it become a lifesaving diet. I know of one individual, Joe, who had open heart bypass surgery twice, had multiple coronary artery stents, was on maximum drug treatment, and continued to have chest pain with only minimal activity and demonstrated apparent progressive disease.

Joe's cardiologist basically told him to get his affairs in order because there was nothing else that could be done to help him. This person was a very bright former college professor who was not willing to throw in the towel. He studied all forms of radical treatments for coronary heart disease. He came upon Esselstyn's work at Cleveland Clinic and decided he had nothing to lose by trying his diet. He went on this extreme diet, and within a few weeks he was able to walk on the treadmill without pain. At this time as I finish the writing of this manuscript, he is still on this planet. It has been six years since he placed himself on the doctor's diet.

Should we all be on this very strict low-fat diet? I feel the answer is no. Good randomized controlled trials have shown that supplementing one's diet with olive oil and nuts lowers the risk for atherosclerosis.[18] Also observational studies have shown that diets containing fish result in lower cardiovascular disease.[19] The other major factor is that the body needs fats. Essential fatty acids have many uses in the body. With deficiencies in these fats, a person can have skin conditions such as scaly dermatitis, hair loss, and decreased platelets, which are involved in blood clotting. With lack of these fatty acids a person has the potential for fat-soluble vitamin deficiencies. Those are vitamins K, A, D, and E. Some parents become so extreme in their push to not only have this extreme low-fat diet themselves, they also place their own children on these diets. With such a restricted low-fat diet, there is the potential for children to have their growth and cognitive and visual functions to be negatively affected.[20]

When fat was said to be the villain robbing us of good health, people changed their diet and began to prepare more high carbohydrate foods. Pasta, rice, and various other grains became the main dishes for dinner instead of meat.

With this trend to eliminate fats, all kinds of low-fat, processed junk foods also flooded the market. These foods were loaded with refined carbs and high-fructose corn syrup. Unfortunately, with these types of carbs instilled into our diets, there was actually a higher risk for heart disease, diabetes, and obesity. They were all the diseases that the low-fat diets were meant to treat.

The Introduction of Low-Carb Diets to Solve the Dangers of Eating Excessive Carbs

Then in 1972, along came Dr. Atkins with his book, *Dr. Atkins' Diet Revolution*, to rid the world of the ubiquitous terrible carbs. One of the real advantages of this low-carb diet, according to Dr. Atkins, was that it decreased a person's appetite. I have to admit this is a common theme of my patients who have committed themselves to this diet. When you eliminate carbs you have only proteins and fats left. Diets high in fats have a slower rate of digestion. With a slower breakdown of food, food is absorbed more slowly, and a person doesn't have spikes in insulin. These spikes of insulin have a significant effect of increasing a person's appetite.

When we get rid of carbs we need to look for tastier foods. One of the worst results of this is that one of the most commonly eaten foods on the low-carb diets is cheese. Every person at a cocktail party loves cheese, but unfortunately our bodies don't. A very good book, *The Cheese Trap*, by Neal Barnard, MD, discusses why.

The processing of cheese causes the following:

1. Processing of a cheese product results in a concentration of calories. A cup of milk has 149 calories; a cup of melted cheddar has 986 calories.

2. It also concentrates dairy proteins, particularly casein. For some people, these proteins trigger respiratory symptoms, migraines, arthritis, skin conditions, and other problems.

3. It concentrates cholesterol and saturated fat, often causing a person's LDL to elevate, which increases the risk for vascular diseases and Alzheimer's.

4. Most cheeses have a high salt content, which increases the risk for hypertension.

5. The reason for the high sodium is that it stops bacteria from growing inside the cheese and improves the texture and enhances taste. And, most importantly, salt is added for safety reasons since it acts as a natural preservative.

The high levels of fat, whether it is cheese or some other form of fat, can slow your metabolism. When you eat fatty food, some of that fat works its way into your muscle cells. As it builds up, it interferes with the cells ability to produce mitochondria. Over time it reduces the number of mitochondria in your cells. The mitochondria are the major energy producing organelles of cells. By increasing fatty foods, as stated by Dr. Barnard, your metabolism slows down. This ultimately makes it more difficult to burn calories. A study done looking at muscle biopsies on individuals on a high-fat diet showed that in only three days there was a slow down when the genes began producing mitochondria.[21] It appears that saturated fats are worse in this regard than unsaturated fats.

At Virginia Tech they had a similar observation. In their research kitchen volunteers were divided into two groups. One group was given a diet that contained 55 percent of the calories from fat, and in the second group 30–35 percent of its calories were from fat. After five days, the researchers took samples of the muscle cells of both groups and found that those individuals eating 55 percent of their diet from fat compared to those volunteers eating 30 to 35 percent of their food from fat were less able to metabolize calories.[22]

Extreme Low-Carb, High-Fat Diets

Another very popular low-carb diet is the ketogenic diet. This diet consists of a very low-carb, high-fat diet that shares many similarities with the Atkins and other low-carb diets. It involves drastically reducing carbohydrate intake and replacing it with fat. The reduction in carbs puts your body into a metabolic state called ketosis.

The theory is that when this happens, your body becomes efficient at burning fat for energy. It also turns fat into ketones in the liver, which can supply energy for the brain. Ketogenic diets have been shown to reduce blood sugars and insulin levels.

There are different versions of this diet. The standard version is a very low-carb, moderate-protein, and high-fat diet. It typically contains 75 percent fat, 20 protein, and only 5 percent carbs. This has become a particularly popular diet with individuals trying to prevent diabetes.

There has been some anecdotal evidence that suggests the ketogenic diet may be helpful with some patients having memory loss from Alzheimer's. It became popular when it was realized that Alzheimer's patients often lose their insulin receptor sites on the brain.[23] These are the sites that insulin deposits glucose for the brain to use for energy. Without a location for the insulin to relinquish its glucose, the brain cannot use its basic fuel source, glucose. The cells without this basic energy can be seriously injured or die. With a ketogenic diet the body has fatty acids that float around that can be used by the brain for energy. The research on this is still limited.

Finally the real reason that the majority of people will choose either a low-fat or a low-carb diet is to lose weight. Therefore the big question is which diet is actually better to lose weight? Low fat or low carb? As it turns out the answer is both have the same effect. A recent study done at Stanford showed that both diets of low fat and low carbs were equally effective in losing weight. There was no statistically significant difference between the two groups over a twelve-month time frame.[24]

THE MODERATION APPROACH TO HEALTHY EATING

1. Consider an extremely low-fat diet like what Esselstyn proposes if you have significant atherosclerotic vascular disease.

2. If you or a loved one has Alzheimer's you may want to consider a trial of a ketogenic diet.

3. If there is a strong family history of diabetes, or you yourself are having signs of prediabetes (see insert below),

consider a diet lower in carbs especially concentrated carbs like sweets and starches.

IIIIIIIIIIIIIIIIIIIIIIIIIIIIIIIIIIIIIIIIIIIIIIIIIIIIIIIIIIIIIIIIIIIIIIIIIIIIIIIIIIIIIIIIIIIIIIIIIIIIIIIIIIIIIIIIIIIIIIIIIIIII

Prediabetes, also called metabolic syndrome, is diagnosed if a person has 3 of the following 5 things:

a. Increased waist size (>38 in. for men and >35 in. for women)

b. Triglycerides >150.

c. Fasting blood sugar above 100 (if >125 you are already a diabetic)

d. Elevated blood pressure.

e. Low HDL cholesterol (men < 40 or women < 50).

IIIIIIIIIIIIIIIIIIIIIIIIIIIIIIIIIIIIIIIIIIIIIIIIIIIIIIIIIIIIIIIIIIIIIIIIIIIIIIIIIIIIIIIIIIIIIIIIIIIIIIIIIIIIIIIIIIIIIIIIIIIII

4. Keep in mind that the types of fats and carbs in your diet are just as important as the percentages of each group in your food.

5. Avoid saturated fats that come from butter, cheeses, and animal fats.

6. Avoid trans fats, if they are still around.

7. Limit the quantity of Omega 6 oils like sunflower and safflower oils. They have the potential of causing increased inflammation in the body.

8. Increase Omega 3 fats in your diet which are from the nonpredatory fish and plant oils like walnuts.

9. Eat carbs that contain high fiber, like whole fruits and vegetables.

10. Avoid the simple carbs that break down to sugar rapidly that you find in sweets, cakes, potatoes, sticky rice (sushi rice), and breads.

11. The basic diet I recommend is essentially a Mediterranean diet. The ratio of fats, carbs, and proteins should be approximately 25 percent fat (mostly monounsaturated fats like olive oil and avocados), 50 percent carbs, and the rest proteins that are plus or minus 5 to 10 percent with each one.

12. If your focus is purely to lose weight, there is no advantage of one over the other when comparing low-fat to low-carb weight loss programs.

Vitamins, Minerals, and Other Dietary Supplements

Are there any I should take regularly?

I am a family physician who is subspecialized in a field of medicine called integrative medicine. This subspecialty began in the 1990s when people were using more and more alternative medicines. In 1997 a study done by Dr. Eisenberg at Harvard[25] showed that 42 percent of the US population were using alternative therapies for nutrition and general health. The number one alternative therapy used at that time in the United States was vitamins and other dietary supplements. They were being advertised on TV and in print. The usage of vitamins, minerals, herbals, and other supplements had become so commonplace that many people no longer considered this to be alternative therapy. There seems to be a vitamin or nutrition supplement for almost everything from improving brain-power, boosting your energy, helping you sleep, making your skin and hair better, to male organ enhancement. These vitamins are touted to make you feel and act younger and to prevent disease. The list is almost endless as to all the possibilities that those wonderful pills can create for you. Advertisements for these products show young healthy adults bouncing across the TV to get you to believe that what they are offering has almost magical effects.

When I began working at Canyon Ranch in 2004, the use of vitamins and other supplements in the average diet was at its peak. We did extensive blood and urine analysis to determine the needs for these. We then recommended multiple vitamins and other supplements at that time. Because of the results of recent scientific studies that have been published in the past fourteen years, I have recommended far fewer dietary supplements then I did when I started here at Canyon Ranch in 2004. We are now going back to the pre-supplement times in our belief that nothing is healthier than eating a well-balanced diet full of fruits and vegetables and the right kinds of carbs and fats. One of the many advantages of a diet of fruits and vegetables and nutritious foods versus taking pills full of vitamins and minerals and other supplements is that the whole foods contain fiber and other less well-defined nutrients. That is not to say that there aren't exceptions to that philosophy, and this will be discussed later in this chapter.

In my subspecialty of integrative medicine, part of the training is to have a good knowledge of supplements. It is important to know that they are called supplements for a reason. They are to augment our meals by filling in the gaps where important nutrients may be missing. They are not to be "the" meal or to be piled onto a "normal" diet for extra nutrients. Just because a little is good, a lot is not necessarily better. I know so many people that go to health food stores selling dietary supplements and walk out with bags of pills. I am not here to discourage you from using vitamins, minerals, and herbs or other supplements. But I am here to educate you on how to make intelligent choices if you decide to take dietary supplements.

Vitamin Supplementation

Vitamins are usually the most common supplements considered. There are times when people are required to take certain vitamins because they have been diagnosed with a vitamin deficiency.

Vitamin B12 Deficiency

"Pernicious anemia" is a medical malady occurring mainly in older people. It was given this frightening name before it was known to be caused by a lack of vitamin B12, and doctors had no way to treat it. Fortunately it is now quite simple to treat with injections of B12.

This condition occurs because some individuals lack a certain hormone in the body called "intrinsic factor" that is needed to absorb Vitamin B12 into the body from the stomach. If a person lacks intrinsic factor, they will have a deficiency of B12. Just taking more B12 vitamin pills orally won't help. The treatment needs to bypass the stomach. This can be done by giving the patient an intramuscular injection of B12 on a regular basis or prescribing a B12 supplement that can be absorbed directly into the bloodstream by placing it under the tongue. Either way the individual needs to supplement their B12 or they will be deficient in this important vitamin.

Deficiencies in B12 can have grave consequences. One affliction is a particular type of anemia called macrocytic anemia. Anemia is a medical condition in which the blood is low in normal red blood cells. B12 is needed to make healthy red blood cells. When B12 is lacking in your body, the red cells produced are abnormal, and they don't function as well.

B12 is also needed for a healthy nervous system. Lack of B12 can be one of the causes of dementia, weakness, fatigue, sensory ataxia (balance problems), and paresthesia (a numbness and tingling of a person's extremities).

Vitamin B9 Deficiency

Vitamin B9 is folic acid, another very important vitamin that is necessary for making new red blood cells. If you have too little, you are said to have a folic acid deficiency anemia.

If you are female and child-bearing age, especially if you are considering having children or could get pregnant, please take 400 mcg of folic acid daily. There is a definite causality between low folic acid levels and congenital neuro-tube defects like spina bifida. The risk of the fetus developing this congenital defect is significantly reduced by simply taking 400 mcg of folic acid daily.

Vitamin D Deficiency

Another important vitamin that is often lacking in the general population, which I talked about at the beginning of this book, is vitamin D. The majority of my patients are low in vitamin D. This is due to the fact that the only natural way to receive vitamin D is from the sun. Everyone is told to stay out of the sun because of the increased risk of skin cancer. If we are exposed to the sun we cover ourselves up with all kinds of clothing or soak our skin with suntan lotion. This is done to prevent premature aging or skin cancer which comes from sun exposure. When we do this, the sun's rays cannot penetrate our skin to make vitamin D. I recommend to my patients to check a vitamin D level. More often than not their levels are low, even with my patients who live in sunny Arizona.

The Daily Multiple Vitamin

Do we all need a daily multiple vitamin? When I was growing up, at my breakfast table every morning was a glass of orange juice and a One A Day multiple vitamin. I couldn't get up from the table until I swallowed my pill and drank my orange juice. I no longer take that One A Day multiple vitamin or any multiple vitamin pill. The literature of the studies about its health benefits just doesn't seem to back it up. Overall data on total mortality rates for those individuals using a multivitamin, showed neither an increase risk or a lower risk compared to the groups not taking a daily multivitamin.[26] Of course there are exceptions to every rule, and at times I will recommend a multivitamin. These are cases when I know the individual is eating poorly or has some form of malabsorption across their gut. Examples of this can occur with the elderly when they are eating poorly or with alcoholic patients who because of their excess alcohol intake will not absorb many of their needed nutrients.

Be Cautious About Taking Vitamin A

Vitamin A is known to be important for healthy skin and a strong immune system. A deficiency of it can result in night blindness, infertility, delayed growth, and respiratory tract infections, and poor healing of wounds, and acne. However, in developed countries it is rare to find people with vitamin A deficiencies. This vitamin is readily available in many fruits and vegetables as well as milk products, eggs, and fish. Vitamin A1 (retinol) is available in meats.[27]

In the US there have been more concerns about the health dangers of taking supplements of vitamin A without an indication that there is a need for this. When the body has excess vitamin A, it is stored in the liver. This can become toxic and cause problems with vision, abnormalities in our bones and skin, and cause cardiovascular problems.[28]

Some studies have shown that there may be an increased risk of osteoporosis with a high dietary intake of vitamin A.[29] Other studies conclude that regularly taking high-dose vitamin A may increase cardiovascular mortality[30] and Beta-carotene (found in Vitamin A) appears to increase the risk of lung cancer in adults who have had smoking exposure.[31]

When Taking Food Supplements Makes Us Ill

It's important to know that dietary supplements can have very serious side effects just like prescription medication. I have seen many patients over the years who were taking combinations of multiple herbs, vitamins, minerals, and amino acid products, who developed serious medical problems from ingesting these chemicals.

An example of this was my patient Jane. She came to visit me because she wanted a second opinion on the syndrome she was suffering from that had been diagnosed as fibromyalgia. These patients have terrible, debilitating muscular pain. It is not a terminal illness but causes great pain and disability. Traditional Western medicine has not been very successful in treating this syndrome. The only thing offered to these patients is antidepressants, pain killers, and neuroleptics. (These are medicines that are used to treat seizures and therefore are used to calm down excitable nerves associated with pain).

The medicines she took helped to mitigate the pain but were are not effective in curing the problem. For that reason, it is very common for people who are suffering from this illness to look for alternative therapies to treat their pain. They will go to multiple alternative-care practitioners looking for some type of answer for their pain. One area commonly explored for treatments is dietary supplements and herbal medicines.

When I saw Jane for the first time, she told me she had been suffering from the pains of fibromyalgia for many years. When she came into my room she was carrying a large grocery bag. When I asked her what was in the bag, she told me it was the vitamins and other supplements she was taking to treat her fibromyalgia. It was filled with nearly thirty jars of different products. I have no idea how she made time during her day to take all those pills. Many who are taking supplements think that because they are "natural" vitamins or herbs they can cause no harm. The sad thing is that in spite of all the pills she was taking, she had little relief from her pain. I asked if I could do some blood studies on her, and she agreed.

When a person ingests these vitamins and other supplement products they have to be biochemically broken down by the body. The two major organs involved in this detoxification are the liver and the kidneys. These organs generally do a good job at this unless they are overwhelmed with multiple chemicals to detoxify. This turned out to be the case for Jane. This overload can result in organ injury, which may be temporary. It can also cause permanent damage. We now know that up to 20 percent of hospital drug-related liver injuries are caused by consumption of dietary supplements.[32] In my concern for the potential ill effects that could have resulted from all the vitamins and herbs Jane was taking, I ordered blood work to look at kidney and liver function.

The next day her blood tests came back showing very elevated liver enzymes. There is always a turnover of cells throughout our body. The liver cells contain enzymes that are involved in the detoxification process. Because of continual cell turnover, there are always some enzymes flowing into the bloodstream. However, if there is an injury to the liver, there will be an excess of cell breakdown resulting in a large amount of enzymes in the blood. Elevation of her liver enzymes meant that her liver was severely injured by all the various supplements she had taken.

I immediately made sure she stopped all her dietary supplements. A repeat blood test two weeks later showed a significant improvement of her liver. Jane was lucky. Her liver was able to recover by just stopping the consumption of all those vitamins, herbs, and other supplements. There are some individuals who are not that fortunate. A seriously injured liver can progress to liver failure.

What Does Vitamin C Do?

Vitamin C is the chemical ascorbic acid, and it is common knowledge that the lack of this essential vitamin causes the terrible disease of scurvy. The discovery of vitamin C in the 1930s by Albert Szent-Györgyi was the basis of modern nutrition and earned him the Nobel Prize in Physiology.[33] Vitamin C is vital to the proper functioning of all of our organs.

In our age, disease from deficiency of vitamin C is seen much less frequently in the populations of developed countries that do not suffer from vast malnutrition and who consume enough fresh produce. The main risk factors for developing a vitamin C deficiency in adults in the US are conditions that cause a poor diet, such as alcoholism or having anorexia or a severe mental illness.[34]

When I was growing up, Linus Pauling was a famous Nobel Prize-winning Laureate who was awarded two undivided Nobel Prizes. In 1954 he was awarded the Nobel Prize in Chemistry. Eight years later he was awarded the Nobel Peace Prize for his opposition to weapons of mass destruction. He became in many ways even more famous for publicly pushing and informing the world that we should all take high-dose vitamin C. He felt it was the cure for multiple diseases and that consumption of vitamin C would prevent you from getting a cold. This is where all the hype associated with taking vitamin C came from.

Since Linus Pauling made his vitamin C claims, it has been extensively studied, especially in the treatment and prevention of infection, most notably the common cold. A review of multiple studies on this topic showed that the administration of vitamin C does not decrease the average incidence of colds in the general population; yet it halved the number of colds in physically active people. Regularly administered vitamin C does seem to shorten the duration of colds. The other important aspect of the vitamin C research is that one has to take high doses of Vitamin C to have an effect.[35]

It should be noted that there are two major problems with taking a high dosage of vitamin C. This has been shown to increase the risk of kidney stones[36] and is often a source of severe diarrhea.

Mineral Supplementation

Iron Deficiency

The macro-mineral iron is a major component of our blood cells. It is needed in our blood stream to make the protein hemoglobin that carries oxygen to our body tissues.[37] A deficiency of iron is the most common cause of anemia that affects around 27 percent of the human population worldwide. Low levels of iron can be caused by poor nutrition or kidney disease or other gastrointestinal diseases or syndromes that cause the loss of iron in our system. Iron deficiency in young children has long been linked to poor cognitive performance, and it is well-known that low levels of iron can affect pregnancies and the brain functioning of the elderly.[38]

A diet that includes regular servings of either red meat, organ meat, seafood, legumes, and dark green leafy vegetables will for most people fill their requirement for iron consumption.[39]

However, young children, vegetarians, menstruating women, and young pregnant women are especially at risk of having an iron deficiency. A person with symptoms of feeling fatigued and weak, or who experiences shortness of breath, dizziness, pale skin, irregular heartbeat, cold hands and feet, or a swollen tongue, should be tested for iron levels. If they are too low, it would be appropriate to add iron supplements to their diet.[40]

But we should never take an iron supplement unless we have received a diagnosis that we are deficient in iron. If we have too much iron in our bodies this also can very dangerous to our health.

Magnesium Deficiency

The macro-mineral magnesium is vital for many bio-chemical functions in our body. The level can become low if people are not eating enough or if they have a condition like alcoholism. A long-term gastrointestinal problem that causes protracted diarrhea can also cause a lack of magnesium. People can also be at risk for this mineral shortage if they take medications that have a side effect of increasing the excretion of magnesium from the body. This will cause a syndrome of "malabsorption," meaning that their intestines do not absorb nutrients properly.

Noticeable symptoms of illness from not having the right levels of magnesium in your body include a lack of energy, light headedness, fatigue, weakness, nausea and vomiting, heart arrhythmias, muscle spasms and cramps, tremors, numbness, and lack of appetite.[41]

In chapter 11, when I discuss digestive disorders, I talk extensively about the problem of a loss of magnesium for PPI medications. If you are taking these drugs to cure your digestive problems, please be sure to have your levels of magnesium tested. Your doctor may then tell you to eat a diet with foods with high levels of magnesium or even suspend your medications to restore normal levels of magnesium in your body.

Magnesium is abundant in the foods we eat. Dark green vegetables, fruits, legumes, whole grains and cereals, sea foods, meats, and milk products all have magnesium. Broccoli, asparagus, beets, bananas, whole wheat, cooked oatmeal, black beans, regular milk, and fish are good sources of magnesium. Nuts and seeds and peanut butter are excellent sources of magnesium. So, apparently, is dark chocolate.[42]

A food problem often discussed in our time is the fact that our produce is often grown in over-farmed soils that do not have the same levels of good nutrients of the food of earlier generations. It is possible that the vegetables or fruits, etc., we depend upon for our magnesium, iron, and other minerals and vitamins are inadequate.

If a patient's repeated blood tests reveal a low level of magnesium in the blood, an oral supplement will likely be prescribed by the person's doctor. It can also be injected into a muscle or vein.

Iodine Deficiency

Iodine is essential for the normal functioning of our thyroid gland and the production of thyroid hormones that determine our bone and tissue growth, brain development, and rate of our metabolism. But iodine deficiency affects about one third of the World's population.

An enlarged thyroid gland (called a goiter) is the most apparent symptom of an iodine deficiency. This might be accompanied by weight gain, an increase in heart rate, shortness of breath. Many health problems can occur in infants and children who have a severe lack of iodine, including a higher rate of neo-natal and infant death, intellectual and neurological disabilities, and other development abnormalities. A pregnant woman needs to be sure she has adequate levels of iodine. Prenatal vitamins that have the recommended dose of iodine and other minerals and vitamins are often prescribed.

Some countries, including the United States, manufacture iodized salt that has greatly alleviated the extent of iodine deficiency.

One of the best sources of iodine in our food is seaweed. Other good sources are fish, plain yogurt, and eggs. But if our soil lacks sufficient iodine because it has been depleted from too much farming, the food that grows there will also be low in iodine.[43]

If a lack of iodine is suspected in a person's diet a doctor may recommend supplementation in the form of potassium iodine and a change of diet.

The Use of Calcium with Vitamin D to Prevent Bone Loss

What about the popular trend of taking a supplement of calcium and vitamin D? Postmenopausal women have a significant risk for getting osteoporosis. Estrogen is very important in maintaining healthy bones. When the estrogen production is suddenly turned off with menopause, bone loss starts. One treatment over the years has been supplemental calcium and vitamin D. When I started working at

Canyon Ranch in 2004 all my postmenopausal patients were advised to take 1500 mg of calcium citrate spread out during the day. In addition, we suggested a minimum of 1000 IUs of vitamin D daily.

I have generally advised women to take 500mg of supplemental calcium and then try to get another 500 mg from their diet. With men, unless they had osteoporosis, I generally don't recommend supplemental calcium. If they do have bone loss, I would generally advise a maximal of 500mg a day. What happened for me to want to make this change? Once again the extremes get you in trouble. Not having enough calcium and vitamin D was thought to increase the risk for bone loss and osteoporosis. But taking too much increases the risk for kidney stones and organ failure, and it also increases the potential for coronary artery problems.

Today the exact dose of vitamin D recommended is poorly understood or agreed-upon, and the recommended dosages for supplementation amounts may soon be changed.

The major forms of calcium supplements are calcium carbonate and calcium citrate. Most individuals who choose a calcium supplement take it in the carbonate form because it is the least expensive. Calcium is broken down to its elements by hydrochloric acid which is produced in the stomach. Of the two types of calcium pills, calcium carbonate and calcium citrate, the calcium citrate is easiest to break down in a low acid environment. For that reason, for individuals that produce less acid in their stomachs, which are often people older than fifty or those who take medication that lowers the acid in the stomach like proton pump inhibitors (example: omeprazole) or H2 blockers (drugs like cimetidine and ranitidine), I recommend calcium citrate.

With vitamin D, the best way to determine if you should take it as a supplement is to have your doctor check your blood level for this vitamin. Your doctor can determine from this information whether or not you are deficient. If your testing shows below normal levels, the doctor can recommend a specific amount of vitamin D to take. I am always fooled by who should and who should not take supplemental dosages of vitamin D. I have seen people that have obviously been frequently out in the sun that have low vitamin D levels and individuals that have stayed out of the sun who have a normal level of vitamin D. The moral of the story is to check your blood levels for vitamins if a deficiency is suspected and then decide if a supplement seems the best choice for you.

Great Caution Should Be Used When Choosing to Take Nutrition Supplements

As I've said, people go to the health food stores and pharmacies to find those magical vitamin, mineral, and other food supplements for many reasons, and that often have been recommended by someone. Many hope that these pills and powders will be their new fountain of youth or help them deal with ailments their doctors have been unsuccessful in treating. And some do hit upon something they find to be very helpful. Just be wary about their potential to harm as well as help.

THE MODERATION APPROACH TO THE USAGE OF DIETARY SUPPLEMENTS

1. For the majority of us, unless you are suffering from an ailment, the need for supplementation is infrequent.

2. We don't need to take a multivitamin unless we have an absorption problem or drink too much alcohol.

3. Beware of taking too much of the fat-soluble vitamins, K, A, D, and E.

4. Ask your doctor for a test of your vitamin D blood level before starting vitamin D to be sure you actually need

supplementation. If your blood test showed low levels for this vitamin and you decide to take a vitamin D supplement, be sure to have a recheck of your blood level one to two months after starting it. You can then determine if you are taking the correct amount.

5. If are over the age of fifty or taking an acid-suppressing medication and you are taking a calcium supplement, make sure it is in the form of calcium citrate.

6. Women who are of childbearing age and have the potential of being pregnant should discuss with their doctor whether they should consider taking folic acid daily to prevent any neural tube defects of the fetus. Taking 400 mcg of folic acid once a day, beginning at least one month prior to conception and continuing this throughout pregnancy, is the recommended dosage.

7. You can get essentially almost all the nutrients and vitamins you need to be healthy from an excellent, balanced diet filled with fruits and vegetables.

5

Alcohol

What about the positive effects from drinking?

Sooner or later you knew I was going to get to alcohol. This is a big open pit, but it needs to be addressed. Every day I am asked by my patients whether or not alcohol is bad for their health. If they do drink, they constantly ask me what is too much. The majority of patients who are asking me how much is too much, are more often than not having too many alcoholic drinks every day.

The subject of alcohol consumption is a classic discussion about moderation in health. For years we have heard from the scientific world that alcohol, especially red wine, is good for the heart. So, should we all be drinking a certain amount?

Let's step back and look at alcohol and how it affects us. There is a major difference in health effects as far as the extremes in alcohol usage. Excess alcohol has no real good outcomes, whereas the other extreme of abstinence has positive effects on the body.

Let's first look at potentially positive effects of alcohol. There have been several studies that show light to moderate alcohol consumption results in a 40 to 70 percent decreased risk of cardiovascular disease compared to abstinence or heavy alcohol consumption.[44] The magic numbers that have floated around the medical world, as far as what is a healthy consumption is one drink a day for women and one to two drinks a day for men.

It was shown that coronary artery disease was decreased, but what about actual mortality? When this was also studied, it was determined that the risk for total mortality was decreased 18 percent when drinking one or two alcoholic drinks a day compared to no alcohol consumed or excess consumption. It is actually a "J" shaped curve indicating no alcohol consumption shows an increased risk of mortality versus having one to two drinks a day. Then beyond this, the statistical level of mortality goes up and continues to go up as consumption increases.[45] The benefit of alcohol seems to have the highest potential effect in women who have a high risk for cardiovascular disease and are over the age of fifty. In women as the consumption of alcohol increases above the light to moderate use to a heavier consumption, the risk of breast cancer and cirrhosis increases. In a large scale study in men there was a decreased cardiovascular disease with light to moderate alcohol consumption. When consumption increases beyond two drinks a day the risk reduction was no longer seen.

One must be aware of how the alcohol is drunk when considering the potential positive effects of alcohol. If a woman drinks a total of seven drinks or a man drinks seven to fourteen drinks spread out over a week time averaging one drink a day for women or one to two drinks a day for men, it has shown to decrease mortality. However, if someone binge-drinks or drinks those seven to fourteen drinks over a few days, it may then have a very negative effect on the person's health, and the mortality risk goes up significantly. Binge drinking is defined as consuming three or more alcoholic drinks in a one to two hour time frame.

Unfortunately I feel this argument for alcohol consumption can be taken too far. There are many psychosocial issues that can arise with the use of alcohol. One of the major reasons we drink alcohol is to relax and loose a little control. This is fine if you are not driving a vehicle, performing at work, trying to get efficient sleep, or making critical decisions. Alcohol can impair judgment and can affect our personal lives if we drink too much at the wrong times. I have seen so many relationships broken up and destroyed because of excess alcohol consumption. As they say, alcohol can loosen the tongue, and with this loss of control, statements and accusations are made that normally would never have been said.

When looking at alcohol in terms of moderation, we can consider that many relationships have been started by a little alcohol. It can benefit individuals who are too shy to meet or say hi to someone and never had the nerve to approach someone they were attracted to. In the right social situation a little alcohol will sometimes break the barrier enough to make the first moves to open a conversation. Alcohol can sometimes give people the ability to loosen up and to relax and be more social, but excessive amounts of alcohol in social situations may also drop one's inhibitions too much. Things might be said that never should have been spoken and can result in a permanent rift in a relationship.

It is important to discuss alcohol if a person is trying to lose weight. As I have often told patients and readers, alcohol contains seven calories per gram, and sugar has four calories per gram. This ends up being a lot of additional calories and added weight. In addition, since we know that alcohol decreases our inhibitions, our will power to keep us from eating that big piece of pie goes right out the window. Even before you get to dessert, if you are having a cocktail or glass of wine before dinner, there are no stops to the pretzels, chips, and cheese that are sitting around asking you to grab and eat them.

Another concern with alcohol consumption is sleep. When I started practicing medicine thirty-five years ago as a country doctor, it was not unusual for doctors to tell their patients to have a glass or two of wine at bedtime if they were having a hard time falling asleep. As incredible as it may sounds now, it was not uncommon for many doctors to also make the same recommendation to pregnant women who were having a difficult time falling asleep! We are now much smarter and realize that the wine mom drinks also crosses the placenta and goes to the fetus. There is no medical consensus about what amount of alcohol is safe to drink when pregnant because the fetus can be very sensitive to alcohol effects at any time , so the recommendation is to not drink during pregnancy.

What does alcohol do to the body in relation to sleep? It is a relaxant and does help a person fall asleep. The problem with alcohol and sleep is that approximately three hours after drinking alcohol a person often gets a rebound phenomenon that either wakes a person up from sleep, or at the very least, prevents a person from getting deep sleep. This ultimately results is dysfunctional sleep, which can lead to daytime drowsiness, increased appetite, weight gain, and potential cardiovascular disease.

Finally let's talk about cancer risk. Unfortunately, in contrast to cardiovascular disease, there is really no lower limit of safety even in light to moderate alcohol consumption. It is dose dependent in that the larger the consumption of alcohol, the higher the risk is for cancer.[46]

WHAT IS THE MODERATION APPROACH TO ALCOHOL?

1. It needs to be very personalized.

2. In general the maximum amount of alcohol to drink for a female should be a one drink a day. For a male the maximum should be one to two drinks a day.

3. We also know that during the first trimester, the fetus is the most sensitive to toxins. Because many women can go several weeks before they know they are pregnant, if

a women is considering becoming pregnant, she should also abstain from alcohol.

4. Binge drinking has no benefit and can only cause harm.

5. If an individual has a personal history of cancer or there is a strong family history of cancer, I would advise less alcohol consumption or even abstinence.

6. If you or your first-degree family members have a history of cardiovascular disease, up to one drink a day for women or one to two drinks a day for men may have some beneficial effect to decrease their risk for heart disease.

7. If you have a history of abuse or addictive behavior, zero alcohol consumption may be a wise choice.

Cleanliness

How clean should we be?

Cleanliness over the last two hundred years has gone from one extreme to another. Until we learned that bacteria were the culprits of diseases that afflicted us, cleanliness basically meant keeping a tidy house.

The Revolutionary Discovery of Antibiotics

Bacteria was first seen by a British microbiologist in 1676, and people learned around two hundred years ago that bacteria were the primary cause of death at that time. This included infectious diseases such as TB, smallpox, cholera, diphtheria, typhus, syphilis, pneumonia, dysentery, and the plague. Contagious diseases remained the leading causes of death in the United States until 1945 when the first true antibiotic, penicillin, discovered in 1928 by Alexander Fleming at St. Mary's Hospital in London, could be produced on a large enough scale to be available to consumers at their corner drugstore. This was the beginning of the antibiotic era that revolutionized the treatment of infectious diseases. Between the 1950s and 1970s many new and novel antibiotics were discovered. After that there have been few new classes of antibiotics, just the many refinements of existing antibiotics.[47]

Sanitation and Disease

But before we had antibiotics, the medical world realized that we could cut down on the number of these infectious diseases by simply keeping things clean.

When I was growing up, my mother was constantly cleaning the house and disinfecting everything because she feared everyone in the house was susceptible to all kinds of terrible infections. Much of this anxiety was brought about by the fact my mother grew up in the 1920s before antibiotics were developed. She witnessed many deaths from transmittable illnesses, especially tuberculosis. She was determined that was not going to happen in her family. She kept everything immaculately clean. She sprayed everything with Clorox bleach, and the house constantly had the faint scent of chlorine.

Ever since we learned that being unsanitary could increase the risk of contagious disease, the general public has been factitious about being clean. When Western civilization pushed to make the environment cleaner, infectious diseases began to decrease significantly. One of the more powerful ways of decreasing infections has been to clean up the water supply. With clean water, waterborne diseases such as dysentery dramatically declined. Another way to reduce morbidity and mortality from infections was to clean up the places that had harbored the most bacteria. This was in hospitals and the operating rooms within the hospitals. It wasn't just a focus on trying to clean away bacteria but on eliminating bacteria altogether. This was accomplished by using stronger and stronger cleaners. These disinfectants had labels saying they killed 99.9 percent of all bacteria and viruses it touched. This significantly lessened the incidence of infections in the hospitals and medical clinics.

Before modern methods of sanitation there were significant infections afflicting both the baby and the mother. Until the last one hundred years infant mortality was one of the most common causes of death throughout the whole human race. And the most common cause of infant mortality was infectious disease. Abraham Lincoln had four children, and only one lived into adulthood. Thomas Jefferson had seven children by his wife Martha, and all but his daughter, Martha, died before the age of five—all were presumed to have died from contagious illnesses.

Complications That Arise from the Goal to Have Clean Environments

Because of the concern about infections, delivery rooms became an extremely clean environment. All the instruments are sterilized, and the delivery rooms are meticulously cleaned with disinfectants. By using these techniques the infant mortality and postpartum infections to the mother precipitously decreased. It would seem logical that if bacterial infections were often a result of unclean deliveries and unsterile environments, and it is a well-known fact that the vagina harbors loads of bacteria, a sterile cesarean should be the best scenario to prevent infant mortality. With this extreme way of thinking, more and more deliveries turned into cesarean sections. In the United States the rate of cesarean delivery (CD) has continued to rise. In 2009 the rate for this was 32.9 percent of all deliveries.[48] This trend is reflected in many parts of the world, with some private clinics in Brazil approaching 80 percent.[49] So what has happened with this increased rate of cesarean deliveries? Should we do more deliveries this way since it is a much more sterile procedure? Once again extremes get us in trouble. Babies born by cesarean sections with sterile environments seem to be having more problems into their adulthood than humans that are delivered through a bacterial-laden vaginal canal.

The sterile environment of a baby born by cesarean section is even more accentuated with the use of antibiotics that have commonly been given to the mother prior to delivery. So what are the consequences of having a cesarean section vs. having a vaginal delivery? The first is that there appears to have more retention of fluid in a baby that has a cesarean section compared to a baby born by vaginal delivery that is literally squeezed through the vaginal canal. Term cesarean section babies have a higher incidence of respiratory distress compared to vaginal delivery because of transient tachypnea of the newborn; this is triggered by excessive lung fluid.

The bigger, and potentially more of a long-term problem, arises from the fact that vaginally delivered babies end up with very different bacteria in their gut compared to the sterile delivery of a cesarean section. This can have significant consequences because the bacteria living in the gut affects many physiologic processes in the body. One effect is an increase of absorption fats from the gut (abnormal bacteria can potentially increase fat uptake) that leads to obesity. Another effect is an influence on our moods (more serotonin is produced in the gut than in our brains), and the ability to have a good immune system can also be influenced by our gut bacteria.

Another difference in the two ways of delivery is that when the infant goes through the birth canal it gathers the vaginal bacteria, and it is ingested and eventually ends up in the infants gut. Babies born from Cesarean section end up with different bacteria that is found on the individual's skin of the health care providers that are caring for the baby. This bacteria is often *Staphylococcal* and *Actinobacteria* vs. vaginally colonized bacteria which is predominantly *Lactobacillus*. Initially one of the advantages of having *Lactobacillus* is that it helps the infant digest milk better. In terms of immunity and the gut bacteria, it has been shown that the bacteria stimulate the lymphoid tissue in the gut, which produces antibodies to pathogens.[50] The bacteria in the gut help support the immune system in attacking pathologic bacteria and leaving the good bacteria alone. This may also help reduce overreactive immune responses that may lead to allergies and autoimmune diseases. There is no question that there is a huge rise in allergies and autoimmune diseases, which may be a result of the increased incidences of cesarean section in addition to the overall obsession about cleanliness.

The "Hygiene Hypothesis"

In medicine this refers to the hypothesis that a lack of early exposure to infectious agents in childhood suppress the development of the immune system and increases the susceptibility to allergic diseases.

An article titled "Hay Fever, Hygiene, and Household Size" that led to the "Hygiene Hypothesis"[51] was originally presented in the *British Medical Journal* in 1989. The author's study showed there appeared to be an inverse relationship between the number of older siblings a person had and the severity of symptoms associated with hay fever. Generally in most households the more older siblings you may have, the less importance there is on keeping things around you clean. This study which showed how exposure to organisms in our environment affects our immune system was subsequently expanded by other researchers beyond hay fever to other allergic diseases, asthma, and atopic dermatitis and autoimmune diseases such as type 1 diabetes, Crohn's disease, and multiple sclerosis. The occurrence of these diseases is higher in more affluent, Western, industrialized countries.

Several theories have emerged that suggest environmental influences are contributing to this phenomenon. Most notably, the "hygiene hypothesis" suggests that an overly clean environment, especially in early childhood, may contribute to the development of several childhood diseases.[52] There was a feeling by the medical establishments during the 60s and 70s that because of the great efforts in cleaning, sanitizing, and antibiotics, that we may be able to eliminate infectious diseases altogether. In 1967 William H. Stewart, MD, the

US Surgeon General, traveled to the White House to deliver one of the most encouraging messages ever spoken by an American public-health official. He said, "It's time to close the books on infectious diseases, declare the war against pestilence won, and shift national resources to such chronic problems as cancer and heart disease." The reason for all this happy hysteria was attributed to the presence of lifesaving antibiotics.

We used to say in medical school during the 1970s that no one should go into the subspecialty of infectious disease. It was felt to be a dying subspecialty. The thinking among the students was that with all the fantastic new broad-spectrum antibiotics that were being produced, anyone could treat infections. You didn't need to bring in a subspecialist to treat infections. As a physician, if you suspected an infection, you just started your patient on one of these broad-spectrum antibiotics that seemed like it could kill almost anything. The majority of these antibiotics were lifesaving to my very sick patients. However, it became evident that there was a severe consequence to the common use of these lifesaving broad-spectrum antibiotics. This has occurred very slowly over years. These broad-spectrum antibiotics, which at one time were able to kill most bacteria, have slowly lost their effectiveness.

Resistance to Antibiotics in an Era of Fierce Bacteria

The overuse of broad-spectrum antibiotics has resulted in the emergence of "superbugs." This is because bacteria have the ability to mutate. An antibiotic may be able to get rid of the majority of a particular bacterium, but because of their ability to mutate, a few bacteria may end up being resistant to the antibiotic being used. With this mutation which is the "survival of the fittest," these new bacteria are then able to live and multiply.

We now have the formation of antibiotic-resistant bacterial infections and are at the brink of a major medical crisis. The hotbed of antibiotic-resistant bacteria has been our hospitals, especially with patients that have several complex medical issues. During their hospitalization these patients are likely to be on multiple antibiotics. Every time they get another infection the bacteria becomes more and more resistant to the antibiotics administered. Their infections are then very difficult to treat, and the mortality for these patients is very high. Unfortunately this dilemma is not only a problem in hospitals and nursing homes. It is now occurring in the community.

When I was in private practice from 1982 to 2004 before coming to Canyon Ranch, I rarely dealt with a superbug called MRSA. It stands for Methicillin (an antibiotic) Resistant Staphylococcus Aureus infection. I only saw this superbug with immune-compromised patients who had been on multiple antibiotics in nursing homes and in hospitals. Over the last ten years I have occasionally helped out at some of the local outpatient care facilities. Whenever I see a patient who presents with a skin abscess, in the majority of cases the causative agent has been MRSA! This superbug, which was resistant to most, but not all, antibiotics, has gone from this rare bug that was seen only with immune-compromised patients in nursing homes or hospitals, to a common community acquired infection.

The other infection that has increased exponentially over the past few years is C. diff. (*Clostridium difficile*). This bug causes a profuse watery diarrhea that can occur after a person has been placed on an antibiotic. The bacteria that causes this disease lives in the intestines but is small in number when all the other bacteria are in the intestines. When the regular bacteria that normally inhabit the large intestine are killed off because of the use of an antibiotic, the C. diff. has room to grow. This causes a severe potentially life-threatening diarrhea.

When I was in my training at the hospital thirty-five plus years ago, we occasionally heard about an isolated case of C. diff. It was originally thought that only one antibiotic, clindamycin, could cause this disease. The fact is, my very first patient I had in private practice that came down with this disease was taking clindamycin for facial acne. The medical term for this C. diff.-causing disease is called pseudomembranous colitis. They gave it this name because when you look into the colon of a patient who has this disease, there appears to be false membranes extending from the wall of the colon. It is not an actual membrane but simply the inflammatory response that occurs with this disease. This once rare disease has now become common. It is now found to occur not only with clindamycin but with many other broad spectrum antibiotics such as fluoroquinolones, cephalosporins, and broad-spectrum penicillins. Unfortunately even the antibiotics that are used to treat this infection like Vancomycin can cause this disease.

Pseudomembranous colitis is just one problem seen with the overuse of antibiotics. Other diseases that are considered mild compared to pseudomembranous colitis are still very uncomfortable. The most common is vaginal yeast infections, which can be seen with women after they have taken an antibiotic. This is such a common problem that many women will ask to be given an antifungal treatment each time they are prescribed an antibiotic.

In order to kill the bacteria, we have been using stronger and stronger antibacterial cleaners. There has been a push to kill all the bacteria that plain soap is unable to kill. Because of this, antibacterial soaps were made. Most over-the-counter antibacterial soaps at one time contained the chemical called Triclosan. Just recently in the fall of 2016, the FDA worked to eliminate this chemical. More specifically, in medical terms, Triclosan was found to be an endocrine disruptor. The concern was that it mimics the chemical structure of a thyroid hormone and therefore blocks the thyroid hormone from attaching to the receptor site. When this happens the person affected can develop the signs of low levels of thyroid hormones. The usage of the hand gels had been so common that a study done in 2008 showed that of all the people that had their urine randomly tested for the presence of Triclosan were found to be positive 75 percent of the time.[53]

WHAT IS THE MODERATION APPROACH TO CLEANLINESS?

1. Being clean certainly has shown to be beneficial. Infections such as tuberculosis and dysentery have significantly decreased along with perioperative and postpartum infections simply by cleaning up the areas of hospitals and other institutions where patients have medical procedures or where they stay and are cared for.

2. Remember that you can decrease incidences of wound infections and the spread of the common viruses by the simple technique of good hand washing with regular soaps that do not contain antibiotics.

3. Keep things clean by using nontoxic cleansers such as vinegar and water and simple soap and water.

4. Keep your drinking water clean by using the recommended treatments for contaminated waters if you have private wells or there is an outbreak of contaminated tap water. This is extremely important in disaster situations like regions following hurricanes or earthquakes. This will significantly decrease the risk of life-threatening diseases like cholera.

5. Try to use antibiotics sparingly. The CDC (Center for Disease Control) recommends the following: Be more discretionary about the use of antibiotics. Do not treat every upper respiratory infection with an antibiotic. The far majority of these infections are viral and do not

respond to antibiotics. If your doctor is concerned that there might be a true bacterial infection, such as one that would be seen in a positive culture, it would then be appropriate to use antibiotics.

6. The other recommendation by the CDC is to finish the complete course of antibiotics. (Please see https://www.cdc.gov/antibiotic-use/index.html) When we don't finish the full course of the antibiotic, it can result in a partial treatment of the infection. This gives the infection the opportunity to return, and it increases the risk of developing an antibiotic resistant bacteria.

7. Unless there are obvious medical reasons to have a cesarean section, like life-threatening events for the fetus or the mother being ill from severe preeclampsia or an uncontrolled maternal bleed (placenta previa), there should first be an attempt to deliver infants vaginally. The hope is that soon the number of cesarean sections will significantly decrease.

8. We don't need to keep our kids in a bubble. They can get dirty. Parents don't have to sterilize everything a baby plays with. The kids that stay clean but are not obsessively sterilized seem to do better and have less allergies as they grow into adulthood. They need to wash their hands and take a shower using soap and water and not antibacterial soaps.

9. We need to be sure we don't go the other extreme of not keeping our environment clean. Remember that outbreaks of cholera, typhoid, dysentery, hepatitis, and other illnesses are a result of unsanitary conditions.

CHAPTER
7

Boundaries

What's wrong with protecting my personal space?

Many self-help books have been written about having personal boundaries. The majority of these books focus on explaining how we need to set up boundaries so we aren't taken advantage of by the people that are surrounding us. Psychologists teach their patients techniques to develop boundaries to protect themselves from the negative or hostile things in their living situation. But much of what has come to be considered personal "boundary problems" originated with the societal value of the importance of being a good multitasker. The "stars" in our daily environment are often successful middle-aged individuals glorified for being super moms or dads and leaders in many endeavors. In these roles they must head up the local committees for their town and school, get their kids to every soccer practice and game, be their children's scout leader or sports team coach, accept extra assignments at work, and take great care of their aging parents and family members that require help.

There is always one of these stars in a group of friends or coworkers who like to boast how they were able to accomplish so many tasks all at the same time. They make people around them feel less worthy because they are unable to accomplish so many tasks. We are led to believe by our peers that multitasking is the norm. We feel we must accept every job that comes along. This happens at home and at work. In time we become overwhelmed, exhausted, and end up accomplishing very little.

In reality, true multitasking is really not possible. A wonderful interview by correspondent Jon Hamilton on NPR Radio's *Morning Edition* on October 2, 2008, addressed this issue. He interviewed the neuroscientist from MIT, Dr. Earl Miller, who studies this area. He pointed out that people can't multitask very well, especially if they are trying to accomplish similar tasks. Usually that area of processing is located in the same area of the brain, and it competes for that space to solve each problem. What Dr. Miller pointed out was that researchers have data proving that humans are not capable of doing many things simultaneously. Instead, what we actually do is to switch our attention from task to task very quickly. Those individuals that feel they are multitasking are only capable of switching between tasks at a higher rate of speed than most people.

There is one additional discussion on multitasking that is causing me great concern. A recent study published in the journal, *Pediatrics*, looked at the effects of media multitasking on children and young adults when using their computers and smartphones. When all the digital devices and smartphone mania began just a few short years ago, initially parents and the medical world were concerned about what kind of affect would it have on our youth. As with human nature and our ability to be desensitized to recurring events, we ignored potential harmful effects from media multitasking because it seemed like everyone was doing it. Safety in numbers!

We have all seen it. Go to a pizza restaurant and look over at a large table of pre-teens and teens. Most are not carrying on a conversation because they are flying through their smartphones going from one site to another and messaging all their friends almost at the same time. Since the brains of children and young adults are still developing, there is urgency to understand the neurocognitive profiles on them from media multitasking. What this article showed is that our initial fears of the effects of media multitasking may have had some merit. The present review showed a growing body of evidence demonstrating that heavy media multitasking showed differences in cognition (e.g. poorer memory), psychosocial behavior (e.g. increased impulsivity), and neural structure (e.g. reduced volume in anterior cingulate cortex, which is an anatomical region of the brain). So it is okay to tell your kids, no matter how loud they scream, to have down time from their computers and phones.[54]

The other end of the spectrum are those individuals who have been guided by their psychologists or books they have read to establish borders to protect their "personal space." Unfortunately, too many have taken this idea to the extreme and have put up walls around themselves that are a mile high. Many individuals become so focused on protecting themselves that they basically ignore the people around them. They commit all their daily efforts to taking care of number one, and with this behavior create the familiar narcissists who are out to care only about themselves.

When it is 5:00 p.m., and they decide they are officially done for the day, these entitled individuals walk out the door and leave behind their coworkers who are forced to take care of all the loose ends that their colleague did not attend to. It seems they only take on assignments that will work into their schedule. They are rigid in everything they do because they feel they must protect themselves from being taken advantage of. This produces a significant amount of animosity between these rigid, privileged individuals and the people around them who must pick up after them.

I once had a coworker who, every single day, walked out at exactly 5:01 p.m.—never once staying beyond that time. For me this always added at least an hour to my day because I had to take care of all her small tasks that she was supposed to have completed. In health care there are certain things that must be done now and cannot wait until the following day to complete. It certainly did not create a happy work environment.

Sometimes these people become so focused on maintaining their rigid systems that they often become stressed out from trying to remain exactly within the borders they set. Their coworkers and family members become so put off by the barriers these individuals have built that it is very difficult for them to have meaningful personal and family relationships.

The terminology of "bending, not breaking" came about in the late 80s early 90s with the Cleveland Browns of the National Football League. At that time they had a defensive unit that prided itself on being the unit that would bend but not break. This came from the fact that a lot of opposing teams marched down the field against the Browns' defensive unit and made a lot of yards. But when it came to the scoring points against the Browns, the other teams rarely did.

Looking at borders in relation to maintaining good health through moderation, I think we need to approach it like the Cleveland Brown defensive unit. You should bend some in order to accommodate your coworkers, family, friends, and work requirements. But don't become so overwhelmed by taking on so many things that you break. This is a fine line, but it's important to recognize and understand when it is best to say no in a polite, caring way.

THE MODERATION APPROACH TO SETTING
PERSONAL BOUNDARIES

1. When taking on tasks for yourself, workers, or family, be sure they are reasonable and not overwhelming.

2. Think twice before adding extra work or volunteerism to your already packed schedule. This is the time to consider setting limits to prevent you from overdoing it and exhausting yourself.

3. Most days you can probably get out of the office close to 5:00 p.m., but if things are piling up, and leaving at this time it will mean extra work for others at your office, consider staying at work for another thirty minutes, and then everyone will be happy.

CHAPTER

8

Meditation

How often, and for how long, should I meditate?

When I was young there was a pervasive view in the general population of the United States that meditators lived only in India, LA, or the San Francisco Bay area, and the only people in our country who habitually meditated were hippies and weirdos that did not work and were always stoned. The majority of us in health care thought it was ridiculous to think that sitting still on a cushion, crossing your legs, and closing your eyes could possibly help your health. Boy were we all wrong.

Today there are many studies that show the tremendous health benefits of meditation. The amazing thing is that nowadays meditation has become mainstream. More and more individuals are learning to meditate every day. But once again we have a tendency to take something that is healthy and beneficial to an extreme. People who start out meditating within a reasonable time frame may begin meditating for longer and longer times and often at the expense of others. They may not be able to complete projects or take care of tasks and therefore others must do it for them. If you are a monk, it's okay because this is part of your daily ritual, but for the rest of us it can definitely create a problem.

I first learned about meditation in 1968 when The Beatles traveled to northern India to take part in an advanced Transcendental Meditation (TM) training course at the ashram of Maharishi Mahesh Yogi. Since The Beatles were one of the most famous Rock bands in the world at that time, this invited widespread media attention. Unfortunately, most of us did not understand what TM was all about, and I, like many others, thought that this Eastern-religion oriented movement had a cult-like feeling about it. It was the time of hippies, getting high on drugs, incense, and free love. Many people, including me, felt it was just another excuse to get high. Aspects of this movement were in every direction you looked. This was the time when posters became popular. In every college dorm there were posters of yogis in meditation poses. But most of my college friends didn't understand what meditation was all about, so we discounted the whole movement.

I was not exposed again to meditation until I became friends with people who had previously lived in Southern California. I found out soon after our friendship began that they practiced meditation twice a day, and each session lasted for a prolonged period of time. I learned not to come by their house or call them during their meditation hours because it was a sacred time for them.

Needless to say, it seemed like we, the non-meditators, were constantly walking around on eggshells trying to prevent an interruption of the meditators. Unfortunately, this resulted in a lot of animosity between the two groups. As meditation became more and more popular for reasons that I will soon disclose, there also seemed to be an air of smugness among those who meditated compared to those that did not follow this practice.

Because I, like many other, people were overwhelmed by the attitudes of those that meditated and the excesses associated with the "true" meditators, this turned many of us off and prevented us from using meditation as part of our lifestyle. This is very sad because people who do not meditate miss out on significant health benefits. The most important thing to know is that to obtain these health benefits you don't need to isolate yourself from the rest of the world for long periods of time to meditate. My point is not to try to prevent someone from meditating for prolonged periods of time but for people to know that if you meditate in moderation for shorter periods you can still gain the benefits that this practice has to offer.

So what are the benefits of meditation? Let's look at some of the recent science associated with meditation. First of all we know that the number one killer in men and women is cardiovascular disease. Therefore anything we can do to decrease cardiovascular disease that is simple, nontoxic, inexpensive, and not time-consuming is obviously a good thing. Meditation fits that bill. Recent studies looking into this have been very promising. These studies have shown that meditation has a significant impact on reducing the risk factors associated with cardiovascular disease. These studies were done on people who meditated for thirty minutes or less a day. The cardiovascular risk factors that were lowered with daily meditation were stress reduction, smoking cessation, and blood pressure reduction; there was also improved insulin resistance, improved endothelial function, and decrease of inducible myocardial ischemia.[55]

The usage of smartphones has made this even easier to measure. A study using a smartphone app for breathing awareness meditation (BAM) was used on pre-hypertensives (defined as a systolic blood pressure of 120 to 140). In as little as five minutes twice a day there was a positive effect in lowering systolic blood pressure.[56]

Meditation has recently been looked at to see if it has benefits for Alzheimer's patients. As we know, Alzheimer's is the most common form of nonreversible dementia. It affects over five million people in this country. Of the ten leading causes of death, it is the only one that until recently had little or no means of prevention. But a study of subjects with cognitive decline and mild cognitive impairment revealed that only a few minutes a day of meditation improved their memory. In addition to this, meditation was shown to improve sleep, decrease depression, reduce anxiety, downregulate inflammatory genes, upregulate immune system genes, improved insulin and glucose regulatory genes, and increase telomerase by 43 percent, the largest ever recorded.[57] All of this with just twelve minutes of meditation a day!

If one has the ability to meditate for long stretches of time, is there any benefit to this? We need to look at the Buddhist monks who are skilled in this practice for answers to this question. The monks have been most extensively studied in the USA at the University of Wisconsin-Madison. Much of the work has been done using functional MRIs. This imaging has shown actual changes in the brain in those who do extended meditation, especially the region of the brain called the amygdala. Their work showed that prolonged activation in this area was associated with a decrease in emotional reactive behaviors. The other really interesting finding was that the monks were able to prevent getting "stuck" on a target. This means that a person can engage and easily disengage on a particular subject matter. Their brains have enhanced focus, memory, learning, and consciousness. At the same time they experience less depression, less anxiety, and less addiction.[58]

Yes, on the surface it may sound wonderful to be able to go about life without depression and anxiety and not need to worry about addictive behavior. However the ability to meditate all day long in a monastery is pretty much out of the question for 99.9 percent of us. Unless we want to isolate ourselves on the top of some mountain, it cannot happen to us for practical reasons. Even if we could carry out hours of meditative practice, life as we know it would be over. Life would be without the highs or lows most of us are accustomed to. This is not the way of life of the rest of the population, and in many ways it could feel like we are living in a world of drones.

These are just a few of the many research studies that have been performed over the last several years showing the beneficial effects of meditation for our health. The other beautiful aspect of meditation is that there is essentially no downside to performing this daily practice. Interestingly, in studies where the practice of meditation had various times needed to perform a daily meditative practice, those individuals who meditated the longest were, not surprisingly, the least likely to maintain the practice.

A MODERATION APPROACH TO MEDITATION

1. Daily meditation of short duration, from ten to fifteen minutes a day, is a simple, easy activity that has huge positive health benefits. It does not take us away from our daily tasks. That ten minutes of meditation a day can help improve your overall mood and decrease your risk for chronic disease.

2. Unless you are a monk or have the good fortune of having excessive free time on your hands, meditating for long hours is generally not practical. I'm not here to discouraged this practice, because the potential health benefits are huge. But it is important to note that meditation is not an all or nothing practice. Just short intervals of meditation can have significant positive effects on your health.

Making Decisions About Diagnosis and Medications for Common Health Conditions

9

ADHD

*What does it mean when a child receives
this diagnosis?*

Growing up in school I remember kids that were fidgety, couldn't sit still, and always seemed to get into trouble. They kept doing things over and over to irritate the teacher or other students. They were continually being reprimanded by their teachers and were constantly yelled at to stay in their seats. They were commonly sent to the principal's office and often even paddled by the principal for their "misbehavior."

When I first started practicing family medicine, the diagnosis given to these fidgety children was hyperactivity. These children were very impulsive and could not sit still or stay focused long enough to read, study, or complete a simple task. They were constantly in motion. This diagnosis later became known as ADD or Attention Deficit Disorder. As physicians we did everything we could do to calm these children down. We kept stimulants such as caffeine away from them. We also told parents to avoid using decongestants which could have a stimulating effect. The other theory put out mainly by parents was that sugar was the cause of this problem. We were not successful in treating these children. We tried behavioral modification with moderate success at best.

Suddenly a theory evolved that giving stimulants actually slowed them down. At that time in the medical world most of us thought this was crazy. We had been treating this problem by trying to eliminate stimulation. How in the world could adding stimulants calm these kids down? Well, for many children it did. The mechanism of the action of stimulants in ADHD is not known, but most likely involves increased intrasynaptic concentrations of dopamine and norepineph-rine.[59] Health care practitioners caring for children finally saw a ray of hope for treating these "unruly" kids.

Let's jump ahead thirty-five years to how the medical profession mainly views this problem now. The term ADHD, Attention Deficit Hyperactivity Disorder, is now one of the most commonly diagnosed chronic illnesses of children. The American Psychiatric Association Diagnostic and Statistical Manual of Mental Disorders, Fifth edition: DSM-5. Washington: American Psychiatric Association estimated in 2016 that 6.1 million children in the US were given this diagnosis. ADHD is then divided into three different types: Inattentive, Hyper-active-Impulsive, and Combined. The Inattentive form is a person who is easily distracted and has a very difficult time focusing and at the same time does not have any signs of impulsiveness or hyper-activity. The Hyperactivity-Impulsive forms of ADHD are individu-als that show only signs of hyperactivity and impulsiveness without signs of inattentiveness. Finally, the Combined category is just that—it's a person who has both inattentiveness and hyperactivity-impul-siveness. The following are the characteristics used for diagnosis of each category:

Signs of the inattentive child:

- Easily distracted
- Forgetful even with daily tasks
- Can't organize

- Can't stay on task like homework
- Doesn't listen to someone who is talking to them
- Can't pay attention to details

Signs of Hyperactivity and Impulsivity:

- Appears to be always on the go
- Talks all the time
- Interrupts conversations
- Has a hard time waiting in line
- Interrupts conversations
- Fidgets all the time in their seat
- Has a hard time remaining in their seat

Children, teens, and now even adults are commonly prescribed stimulants to treat their attention deficit. According to records recorded by the FDA, the amount of stimulants prescribed in this country in 2013 was about 211 tons! Over the thirty-five years as a practicing family physician, I have seen the usage of stimulants increase exponentially. It was pointed out in an article written in the *Huffington Post* by Dr. Lawrence Diller at UCSF that nearly one in five high school boys have been diagnosed with ADHD.

When I started practicing medicine, I rarely prescribed stimulants. Stimulants like Ritalin and Adderall are a class II narcotic, which is in the same drug class as opium and codeine. Because of this, I was quite conservative about prescribing such powerful drugs to these children and young adults.

To medicate or not to medicate is often a big question. In my medical career, as I said, I have seen the extremes on both sides of the dilemma. When I started practicing medicine stimulants were rarely prescribed. As I mentioned, at this time almost one in five teenage boys is diagnosed with ADHD. Are the majority of children in some way impulsive and hyperkinetic? The answer of course is yes. That is the beauty of youth. They have energy to burn. The problem is determining what is just youthful energy and what is actually a pathologic syndrome. A child who can never sit still, is always running around the house, always seems to be in trouble because he or she is constantly into everything and can't finish anything, is an easy child to be diagnosed and worthy of a trial of a stimulant. Many of these children benefit greatly after being placed on stimulants. Their classroom work often improves and they can finally sit long enough to finish a project. Their social skills often improve, and they seem to develop better relationships with their peers. The use of medications may seem like a miracle to both the child and the parents.

When deciding whether or not to use medication to treat this disorder, it is very important to look at the potential side effects that can occur with the use of these stimulants. First of all there are two major classes of stimulants. They are methylphenidates that include Ritalin, which is one of the medications that has been used for years for ADHD, and amphetamines, which includes dextroamphetamine. The frequency of potential side effects is similar in both groups. The most common side effects are anorexia (stimulants have been used for years as food suppressants), poor growth, sleep disturbance, and increase in mood swings and jitteriness. One can also have cardiovascular side effects, which includes elevated heart rate, elevated blood pressure, priapism (a persistent erection), and arterial blood vessels going into spasms. (An example is Raynaud's phenomenon where fingers and toes turn white and blue in cold weather.)

In terms of having a growth disturbance, this seems to decelerate over time and cessation of the medication may result in normalization of growth. Also, minor side effects include headaches, gastrointestinal symptoms, and dizziness.[60, 61, 62]

One extreme is not treating children who have severe forms of ADHD. This can occur when parents decide that all medications, especially stimulants, are bad and they are adamant that their child is not going to take drugs to treat a focus problem. These untreated children that may have serious attention deficit disorders often never reach their full potential in the classroom and struggle most of their lives in social situations.

Unfortunately the other extreme is the overuse of stimulants. According to the FDA, America produces 70 percent of the world supply of amphetamines every year. Amphetamines, legal and illegal, have been around since 1929[63] and have repeatedly found their way into the mainstream culture over the years for use in treating depression, asthma, narcolepsy, weight control, and now attention deficit hyperactivity disorder.

Living in a college town and having my daughter recently graduate from that college, I witnessed first-hand the widespread excessive use of stimulants. These drugs were being used for reasons it wasn't prescribed for. Examples were weight loss, trying to stay awake all night to study for a test, or for finishing a project due the next day. The majority of stimulants are legal prescription drugs initially, however nearly a third of those legally prescribed drugs end up being used illegally.[64]

It is my opinion that one in five teenage boys taking stimulants is excessive. The hormone called testosterone begins to surge at this age, and many of the actions that these boys (and girls) are doing in terms of impulsivity can be attributed to this magical hormone. We must remember there are many potential side effects that can occur with stimulants. Stimulants are a very serious medication. If not taken for exactly what they should be prescribed for, which is a diagnosis of attention deficit, they have a huge potential for abuse. When this happens the person can easily fall into the dangerous roller coaster cycle of feeling down and deciding they must take another dose to get up.

It is important to get an accurate diagnosis before being placed on these medications. As a family physician I have had parents come in to see me to demand that their child be placed on a stimulant because their child was unruly or was not doing well in school. Often the teachers would send notes home with the students telling parents to take them to see their doctor and strongly suggesting their child be placed on a stimulant. Over the years I have heard doctors on the radio say that it was practically malpractice if a child had signs of attention deficit and their doctor did not place that child on a stimulant. Parents were told their child had a chemical imbalance and had to be treated with chemicals.

The other group of patients I saw were parents of diagnosed ADHD children that had met with the pediatric psychologist. During their meeting to discuss their child, the psychologist would refer the parents back to me to be placed on medication because studies determined that when a child has ADHD there was a greater than 40 percent chance the parents also had ADHD. Here we go with the extremes again. Yes, there is absolutely no question a child or adult with a diagnosis of ADHD who is placed on medication may find this is life changing for the better. However, we still need to be more discretionary about placing kids and adults on these drugs. The children especially are then labeled as being "ill" and considered to have something wrong with them. This is reinforced in school when they have to go to the school nurse to get their medication.

I'm often asked whether a child that has been properly diagnosed as having ADHD, can "outgrow" this problem. Actually, there is some proof that this can happen. As a child grows their prefrontal cortex matures as well. This changes their thinking, and often their symptoms may decrease. Approximately one-third of those children diagnosed with ADHD no longer have symptoms of this when they reach adulthood. Many of the remaining two- thirds will have a significant decrease in their symptoms as they reach adulthood.[65]

In summary, if there is a real concern that a child or adult may have significant problem of staying focused or is constantly hyperactive beyond what would be considered "normal," I recommend the following.

THE MODERATION APPROACH TO ATTENTION DEFICIT HYPERACTIVITY DISORDERS

1. Before any medications are prescribed, the person who is thought to have a form of attention deficit needs to go through proper testing by a professional psychologist who specializes in this syndrome.

2. If the diagnosis is made that this individual has ADHD, the first treatment is not necessarily medication but may be a trial of behavioral modifications customized for your child.

3. If the modifications are not effective or are only partially effective, a trial of a stimulant can then be used under the close supervision of a child psychiatrist, psychologist, or a well-qualified pediatrician or family physician.

4. I am a little old-fashioned on this subject, but feel that it's okay to intermittently have drug holidays and to go off the stimulants during weekends or on vacations to see if the child or adult still needs to be on medication.

5. If stimulants are prescribed, the patient needs to be monitored closely by recording and watching their pulse, blood pressure, and weight.

6. Remember that not every child that has some difficulty focusing or is a little overactive needs to be placed on a stimulant.

10

Antidepressants

Why are there so many kinds?
How dangerous are the side effects?

When I started practicing medicine in the early 1980s, very few of my patients were on antidepressants. Only those individuals that had severe clinical depression were on medications for depression. Generally those individuals taking medications were under the care of a psychiatrist who monitored and prescribed them. Since that time, the usage of antidepressants has skyrocketed. Adults in the US consumed four times more drugs for depression in the late 2000s than they did in the early 1990s. Antidepressants are the third most frequently taken medication in the US. Researchers estimate that 8 to 10 percent of the population is taking an antidepressant.[66] 11 percent of Americans age twelve and over are on these medications. Women are more likely than men to take antidepressants and whites are more likely than non-whites to take them.[67] The actual use of medicine for depression began in the 1950s with the introduction of the first two specifically designed drugs for clinical depression: iproniazid, a mono-amine-oxidase inhibitor that had been used in the treatment of tuberculosis, and imipramine, the first drug in the tricyclic antidepressant family.[68] The original antidepressants did help depression. However, they had significant side effects. The major side effect with the tricyclics was fatigue, dry mouth, and weight gain. The major drawback of MAO inhibitors is having many food restrictions. If not followed there is a high potential of a hypertensive crisis.

When I prescribed any of the tricyclic antidepressants, I had to spend a significant amount of time explaining to patients that if they just hung in there for a month a lot of the side effects would go away. Most people aren't that patient, and I really couldn't blame them. More often than not with the older antidepressants, because the side effects were so significant, I would have to start them on a very low dose and then slowly increase the dose over several weeks. For this reason it took a very long time for the patient to get a dosage that had an effective antidepressant effect. Most patients, unless they were severely depressed, gave up on the drugs and decided they would rather be depressed than go through weeks of fatigue, dry mouths, and possible weight gain. Because of this, only the very depressed patients were being effectively treated for depression.

The reason the tricyclic antidepressants have so many side effects is that they block specific receptors called the muscarinic acetylcholine receptors in the body. This can cause a lot of bothersome and potentially life-threatening side effects. These include anticholinergic effects that can affect your heart as well as antihistaminic effects, decreased seizure threshold, sexual dysfunction, diaphoresis (sweating), and tremors.[69] In contrast to some other antidepressants (such as the SSRIs), tricyclic antidepressants can be fatal in doses as little as ten times the daily dose.[70] This toxicity is usually due to prolongation of the QT interval (an abnormal change in the electrocardiogram), leading to cardiac arrhythmias. To complicate this problem, these drugs are fat soluble which means they can hang around a long time in the fat cells and prolong the side effects. This is all of concern to the practitioner who is trying to treat these patients who have severe depression but knows that the medication that they are using has serious potential side effects.

The explosion in the usage of antidepressants began with the group of medications called the SSRIs. That stands for selective serotonin reuptake inhibitors. These drugs prevent the reuptake of serotonin by blocking the receptor sites. By doing this, serotonin levels will increase in the body. Serotonin is one of several neurotransmitters that the body produces (dopamine and norepinephrine are two other major neurotransmitters). When levels of serotonin are low in the body, there appears to be a tendency for the person to have depression. The first in this group of drugs was Prozac. Finally physicians had a drug we could prescribe that appeared to have very little side effects.

Prozac was made by Eli Lilly in the 1970s and was introduced to the public in 1986. All through my residency in family medicine, which had a major focus on psychiatric illnesses, we were taught how to treat severe depression with tricyclic antidepressants such as Elavil. But the large majority of patients that received these antidepressants were given to them by psychiatrists. The general practitioners rarely prescribed them. Now along comes this miracle drug with few side effects compared to the previous generation of antidepressants, and everyone got into the act to prescribe the drug.

The relatively benign side effect profile of the SSRIs is due to their selectivity.[71] None of the SSRIs significantly affect alpha-adrenergic, histaminic, or cholinergic receptors, with the exception of the drug paroxetine, which weakly antagonizes the cholinergic receptor.[72]

Because of the few side effects compared to the tricyclics, other uses were found for the SSRIs besides depression. This included panic disorder, obsessive-compulsive disorder, generalized anxiety disorder, social anxiety disorder, post-traumatic stress disorder, body dysmorphic disorder, bulimia nervosa, binge eating disorder, and premenstrual syndrome.

The pharmaceutical representatives who represented these SSRIs swarmed in on the primary care physicians. They brought in their samples of antidepressant medication to the offices and got access to the doctors by buying lunch for the whole office staff at least once a month and taking the docs out to dinner. They even flew docs to great vacation sites and gave seminars on the favorable effects of their antidepressant drugs.

We in the primary care world were told that these miracle drugs were without side effects. This was also the time when everything you read in the medical journals or was published for the lay public shouted out that depression is a chemical imbalance, and the simple treatment was a drug to correct that problem. People didn't need psychotherapy; they just needed a drug to correct their chemical imbalance. Now with the influx of pharmaceutical reps coming into all the physician offices pushing their new "side effects-free" drugs and the general public getting on board, the pervasive view was felt that no one was supposed to be sad. If you were sad for whatever reason, it was because you had a chemical imbalance. The simple answer to correct this problem was to take this "side effect free" drug to correct your depression problem. Now not only were the psychiatrists ordering antidepressants. Primary care physicians were writing Prozac scripts like candy.

Next the pharmaceutical reps attacked the Ob-Gyn offices and pushed this drug, which is chemically the same drug as Prozac but marketed under the new name, Sarafem. It was used to treat women who suffered from PMS or the emotional ups and downs of menopause. Following this, the cardiologists read studies showing a correlation between post-heart attack depression and the recurrence of heart disease, and they started prescribing these drugs. The other group that started prescribing antidepressants were the gastroenterologists. They had a large group of very difficult patients to treat that were suffering with a condition called irritable bowel syndrome. The consensus was that these patients were all depressed, so they too were given Prozac-like medications. In a relatively short period of time, it seemed like the whole medical world was now prescribing Prozac-like medications.

Other pharmaceutical companies wanted to get in on the money tree and produced their own form of an SSRI drugs. This is when Paxil, Zoloft, and Celexa were made. Each was advertised that it was better than the other. We weren't allowed to be sad. We just needed to take one of these drugs and chemically wash away our depression. The unfortunate consequence of this increased use of antidepressants was that I began to see more and more patients who wanted antidepressants just because they were sad and not because they had clinical depression.

The good news about this antidepressant revolution was that with the increased use of these drugs and the more public acceptance of these drugs, many people were more open about their emotional issues and more apt to seek out help. This was one of the more positive aspects of this group of medications. I saw so many patients who had hidden their mood disorders because of the social stigma that had previously surrounded them. There was no shame in having a heart attack, and everyone in the neighborhood and family members would come and see how they could help them. However, if you had an embarrassing illness of depression, that was not considered socially acceptable and no one wanted to have anything to do with you. Now as a physician it was so much easier to talk to patients about their moods. They became much more open to discussing how they were feeling.

Many individuals were helped with this group of drugs. They finally felt like life was worth living. Also, if one family member had tendencies toward clinical depression, it was likely that other family members had a genuine chemical imbalance. Science showed that this disease was commonly a genetically derived disease. Therefore, if a person was a child or sibling of a chemically depleted person then there was a high likelihood they had this problem and also needed these drugs.

Of course there is no perfect medication for this despite what the pharmaceutical representatives say. SSRIs compared to tricyclic antidepressants have significantly less side effects. However, it does not mean they do not have any side effects. Their effects upon the serotonin receptors can produce unfortunate reactions. They include the following:[73]

- Sexual dysfunction – 17 percent
- Drowsiness – 17 percent
- Weight gain – 12 percent
- Insomnia – 11 percent
- Anxiety – 11 percent
- Dizziness – 11 percent
- Headache – 10 percent
- Dry mouth – 7 percent
- Blurred vision – 6 percent
- Nausea – 6 percent
- Rash or itching – 6 percent
- Tremor – 5 percent
- Constipation – 5 percent
- Stomach upset – 3 percent

The big push to use SSRIs is because they have few side effects compared to other antidepressants. But little is said of the potential withdrawal effects that can occur if a person suddenly stops taking their SSRI. These patients can suffer significant negative physical and psychological effects. Many have the symptoms of:

- Dizziness

- Fatigue
- Headache
- Nausea

Other common discontinuation symptoms include:

- Agitation
- Anxiety
- Chills
- Diaphoresis
- Dysphoria
- Insomnia
- Irritability
- Myalgias
- Paresthesia
- Rhinorrhea
- Tremor

Less common symptoms include electric-like shocks, ataxia, auditory and visual hallucinations, and hypertension. Also, onset of discontinuation symptoms when the drugs are withdrawn typically occur within a few (one to four) days of abruptly stopping antidepressants or tapering them rapidly (i.e. one to seven days)[74] Although these symptoms are usually mild and dissipate over one to two weeks without specific treatment, distressing symptoms can persist for a month or longer, interfere with daily functioning, and may occasionally lead to hospitalization.

Reviews estimate that among patients treated with antidepressants, discontinuation symptoms occur in approximately 20 to 33 percent of them who stop using the drugs.[75]

Once again we must consider moderation in health in dealing with antidepressant medications. Yes, these drugs have been a
godsend to many of my patients. These patients finally got out of
the house and started to engage in social interactions with friends
and family. In some cases it even helped to prevent individuals from
harming themselves. The problem is that not everyone that experiences sadness in their life needs to be placed on medication. There
are a lot of very unfortunate or tragic things that occur in our lives,
like loss and death of friends and family, loss of jobs, divorce, and relationship breakups. It is natural and normal to feel sad. This feeling
can act as part of the healing process that goes on in a person's life.
Some pain and misery, no matter how hard is to go through, helps us
understand how important those losses are to us. Otherwise we may
never have worked so hard in the first place to obtain love or friendship or to do well at something we value. Therefore we in the medical profession need to choose wisely how to help cases when a person
remains sad and unable to engage in daily activities or interact with
other individuals for a prolonged time and can't get out of their hole.
In these instances medications should be considered, and if used the
result may be life-changing.

THE MODERATION APPROACH TO ANTIDEPRESSANTS

1. Sadness is a natural response to bad events that occur in
    a person's life. It is normal to feel down, especially if it is
    a recent event. Some examples are the loss of a loved one,
    loss of employment, or having a medical ailment.

2. Medication should be considered if the depression con-
    tinues beyond a normal grieving time and most notably
    if the person's health is being affected by the depression.

3. SSRIs do have side effects, but they are significantly less than the older antidepressants.

4. Suddenly stopping or rapidly weaning off SSRIs can cause withdrawal symptoms that can make it very difficult to stop these medications. It might take one to two months to wean off SSRIs if you have been on them for a prolonged time.

Digestive Disorders

What are the best treatments, and what are their side effects?

Disorders of the Upper Gastrointestinal Track: Treating Ulcers

During my years of practicing medicine I have seen the evolution in the treatment of excess or relative excess production of acid in the upper gastrointestinal tract. The frequency of these diseases and the treatment of these diseases have changed dramatically over the years since I entered medical school. In medical school in the 1970s, when I was on surgery call, I was frequently up all night with patients with bleeding ulcers. I would constantly run down to the emergency room to see critically ill patients who were vomiting blood because of a bleed from their esophagus, stomach, or the upper part of their small intestines.

These ulcers were formed by an excess production of acid in the stomach. The classic symptoms associated with these upper gastrointestinal diseases are discomfort in the upper part of the stomach. It is usually a burning or gnawing sensation. Ulcers, if prolonged and severe enough, can sometimes erode into a blood vessel. When this happens a bleeding ulcer develops. This can be a serious and even life-threatening problem. We would put a nasogastric tube down through their nose and push ice water down these tubes to try to stop the bleeding.

If it didn't stop, which was quite common, we would need to rush the patient into surgery to open them up to find the actively bleeding stomach or duodenal ulcers and tie it off. Many people died if you didn't get them into surgery in time.

In medical school to make a diagnosis of a nonbleeding ulcer one had to use an X-ray called a barium swallow. You drank down this chalky liquid that tasted awful. As you were drinking this sludge the X-ray technician took X-rays. The idea was for the barium, which is visualized radiologically, to settle into the ulcer pit. It was able to visualize some ulcers, but it missed a lot also. (A few major medical centers were just starting to use the flexible endoscope to look down through the esophagus into the stomach and out into the beginning of the small intestines. This procedure revolutionized the ability to diagnose ulcers.)

Once a diagnosis of an ulcer was made, there was very little I could offer them as a physician to treat them. I would first offer them the always delicious "ulcer diet." This was an incredibly bland diet. You needed to avoid caffeine, alcohol, and spicy foods. You had to eat mild, flavorless food, such as dry meat, plain potatoes, and a few simply prepared vegetables. The only medical treatments we had for ulcers were antacids. Believe it or not some of the older doctors at that time still dripped in continuous milk through a nasogastric tube for the treatment of ulcers!

The Appearance of a Wonder Drug

The year I graduated from medical school, a miracle happened! Cimetidine, initially produced under the trade name Tagamet, was introduced to the public as a prescription drug. It truly was a miracle. This drug is an H2 (histamine) receptor antagonist. Most of us are familiar with the common over-the-counter antihistamines that decrease nasal itching and drainage. Some common antihistamines are Benadryl and Claritin. These block histamine (H1) receptors, which are in the upper respiratory tract. Histamine is the nasty culprit that causes nasal swelling congestion and itching. H2 receptors predominantly line the gut and, when stimulated, increase acid production. Tagamet was the first H2 receptor antagonist that blocked that receptor site and prevented it from being stimulated. This resulted in slowing down acid secretion from the stomach. When patients were put on this medication, ulcers healed much more easily, and many times we were able to prevent ulcers from forming in the first place. This was revolutionary to internal medicine.

Suddenly in the one year from the time I graduated from medical school to becoming an intern, there was an almost eerie quiet during the times I was on surgery call. I actually got some sleep. The emergency room was no longer packed with bleeding-ulcer patients. TAGAMET had arrived! I cannot tell you what a dramatic effect this drug had in medicine. It was the "cure" for ulcers. The drug is still available, and now it is over the counter. It of course was not the perfect drug. It does have its potential problems. First of all, it is short-acting and therefore must be given several times a day. We initially gave it four times a day. Now, it is given twice a day, but probably should be given more often. Also, more recently longer-acting H2 blockers were developed. Two notable ones are ranitidine (Zantac) and famotidine (Pepcid), both of which have replaced cimetidine in popularity.

Proton Pump Inhibitors (PPIs)

After personally witnessing the effects of this miraculous group of drugs, it was hard for me to believe that there were even stronger acid-suppressing drugs to come along. It turned out that while H2 blockers significantly decreased the production of acid in the stomach, there was some development of tolerance to these drugs. They lost some of their effectiveness over time, but they are still remarkable medications. The medical world thought that because of the possibility of tolerance to the H2 receptor and because some individuals still had ulcer symptoms on these drugs, they looked for something stronger. This led the pharmaceutical world in the 1980s to develop what are called "proton pump inhibitors." The first of these powerful drugs to suppress the release of acid secretions in the stomach was omeprazole (Prilosec) in 1988.

||||||||||||||||||||||||||||||||||||||||||||||||||||||||||||||||||||||||||||||||||||||||||||||||||||||||||||||||||||||||||||

THE INTRODUCTION OF PRILOSEC

An interesting, and to some, humorous, story about the introduction of this first new miracle drug in the category of proton pump inhibitors has to do with its original brand name. When Prilosec was first introduced, it was called Losec. This was constantly confused with the medication Lasix, especially when placing telephone orders. Lasix is a diuretic, and these drugs increase the removal of water from our bodies. There were many patients who could not understand why their ulcer symptoms were not going away with this supposedly great drug. At the same time they realized they sure had to go to the bathroom a lot because they were mistakenly given Lasix instead of Losec. Fortunately, it was not long before this problem was recognized and this brand name was changed to Prilosec.

||||||||||||||||||||||||||||||||||||||||||||||||||||||||||||||||||||||||||||||||||||||||||||||||||||||||||||||||||||||||||||

The proton pump inhibitors are the most potent inhibitors of gastric acid secretion available.[76] They block the active secretion of hydrogen ions that causes the acidity. They have been so effective that there was an initial worry that these drugs could cause stomach cancers since stomach cancer often occurs in people whose stomachs have little acid production. We use to limit the use of this drug to only one to two months for this reason. Fortunately, this possible side effect did not occur, and we no longer fear these medications will cause cancer.

The mechanism of action for proton pump inhibitors is that these drugs work by preventing the secretion of acid during digestion of a meal. For that reason they work best when taken before the morning meal. Also it is important to note that it takes several days to get its maximum effect. A 66 percent reduction in acid secretion usually takes five days to be accomplished. H2 blockers, on the other hand, start to work much faster than proton pump inhibitors. Therefore H2 blockers like ranitidine (Zantac) are better for taking care of acute stomach-acid burn. Ultimately over time the H2 blockers are not as effective in lowering overall acid secretion. In comparing H2 blockers to proton pump inhibitors (PPIs), the PPIs are superior in healing peptic ulcers. The PPIs have shown to heal gastro-duodenal ulcers more rapidly than H2-receptor antagonists. A meta-analysis comparing the healing of duodenal ulcers found that 20 mg of Prevacid (a proton pump inhibitor) was superior to Zantac 300 mg a day or 800 mg of Tagamet over a four-week history of treatment.[77]

Gastroesophageal Reflux

Gastroesophageal Reflux Disease, better known as GERD, is caused by the backflow of acid from the stomach up into the esophagus. It can produce many different types of symptoms. The classic symptom is having burning in the mid-chest shortly after eating. Other less subtle signs of excess acid secretion are hoarseness, recurrent cough, and sometimes even new onset asthma has been associated with gastro-esophageal reflux. In the treatment of GERD, PPIs appear to be superior to H2 blockers. It is important to note that unfortunately GERD is often not a curative disease, and a patient has to be given a maintenance therapy to prevent complications of this disease. One of those complications is esophageal strictures, which is scarring in the esophagus. This can result in food getting stuck in the esophagus on its way down into the stomach. This is a major discomfort that puts you in the emergency room. GERD also has the potential for causing a precancerous condition called Barrett's Esophagus. If a person has Barrett's, the rates of getting esophageal cancer are at 0.1 to 0.4 percent per year which is approximately thirty times the risk of the rest of the population.[78]

Overall, the two groups of drugs, H2 blockers and proton pump inhibitors, were found to be effective in treating hyperacidic gastro-intestinal conditions. Everything from stomach discomfort to preventing life-threatening bleeding ulcers seem to respond to these acid-suppressing drugs. Because of the great success rate of treating these conditions, if a patient has any minor symptoms they have been encouraged by their doctors to go on these drugs and to stay on these drugs. Doctors did not want to get called in the middle of the night from patients with ulcer symptoms. It is important to note here that the highest acid secretion in a 24-hour day cycle is right after midnight. That is why many people wake at 1:00 a.m. with abdominal pain and burning that commonly radiates up into the chest. It is not uncommon for patients to feel like they are having a heart attack.

Side Effects from Use of H2 blockers and PPIs

These two drug groups were so successful in treating these hyperacidic states that they were being used more and more. They were even being used for minor acid indigestion. With such excessive usage of these drugs, it was only a matter of time until physicians started to see problems from using these miracle drugs. One of the very first problems that I saw in my practice was an increased risk for developing osteoporosis. One of my jobs at Canyon Ranch is performing DEXA bone density scans to determine bone density. I personally do the scanning and then discuss the results with the patients. I have been observing an inordinate amount of osteoporosis in younger patients. I noticed that a large percentage of those young patients that were being diagnosed with osteoporosis, seemed to be taking proton pump inhibitors on a regular basis. Calcium needs an acid environment to be absorbed across the gut. Therefore, proton-pump inhibitors and H2 blockers, which significantly lower stomach acid secretion, can cause a decrease in calcium absorption. This gets to be an even worse problem when we get older because acid secretion already naturally decreases as we age.[79] A person that has osteoporosis has an increased fracture risk. Hip fractures have been shown to increase in patients who have taken proton pump inhibitors on a long-term.[80] More studies have been done with the PPIs to look further at osteoporosis and fracture risk, but there have also been studies done that show an increased fracture risk with use of H2 blockers.[81]

Another mineral that can be affected by long-term PPI usage is magnesium. Twenty-five percent of those cases that were cited in the study had persistently low magnesium levels despite being given magnesium supplements at the same time. If the PPIs were discontinued, the low magnesium levels could then be corrected with supplementation.[82] As discussed in the chapter on supplements, symptoms associated with low magnesium are fatigue, muscle spasms and cramps, heart arrhythmias, lightheadedness, numbness, and nausea and vomiting.

An important vitamin that can be affected by chronic PPI usage is B12. Vitamin B12, like calcium, is dependent on gastric acid. So if you are continually on a PPI or even a H2 blocker, please check your B12 levels.

Beware of increased risk for unusual infections with chronic PPIs use. Patients whom I placed on a PPI or H2 blockers initially had relief from the classic excess stomach acid secretion, which was a gnawing and burning sensation at the pit of their stomachs. Those symptoms would decrease or go away in about a week. If these patients stayed on the meds for a prolonged period of time (weeks or months), I would occasionally see them come back again with a different type of abdominal pain. It was a bloating and cramping sensation. These same symptoms are commonly seen with individuals with irritable bowel syndrome. This didn't make sense to me at the time. It was occurring at such a high number that it was beyond sheer coincidence. I personally put one and one together and saw the correlation between the usage of PPIs or H2 blockers and the subsequent symptoms of abdominal bloating and cramping. It became such a common complaint that if a patient came into see me with classic irritable bowel symptoms, one of the first questions I would ask is whether or not they were taking a PPI or H2 blocker on a regular basis.

This was also observed by other physicians. Since there was less acid secretion in the stomach there is less ingested bacteria being killed as it entered into the stomach. The result is an excess growth of bacteria in the gut. This condition is called small bowel overgrowth. It is a definite disorder, and it has been studied.[83,84] Some of the newer literature has disputed this previous work and are not as convincing in the correlation between PPI use and IBS.[85] As a practitioner I still ask the question of my patients on PPI use who have IBS symptoms, especially if the IBS it has been going on for a relatively short period of time.

A recent and more frightening potential side effect from prolonged use of proton pump inhibitors in the elderly is dementia. The mechanism of action may be related to the production of Beta-amyloid. Beta-amyloid is the protein deposits that are found in the brains of Alzheimer's patients. In one study looking at mice, PPIs were observed to enhance β-amyloid (Aβ) levels in the brains of mice by affecting the enzymes β- and γ-secretase.[86] The verdict is still out on this and we need more studies to determine the true validity of this potential side effect.

A MODERATION APPROACH TO PPIs AND H2 BLOCKERS

1. Symptoms that are suggestive of excess acid production are burning or gnawing sensation in upper part of the stomach that may radiate up into the chest. These symptoms are usually noted about one half to one hour after eating. This time frame is logical because the highest acid secretion of the stomach is right after a meal because the body is trying to start the digestion of food that was just eaten. The worse symptoms of excess acid secretions are bleeding ulcers. This can be noted in emergency situations in which a person is vomiting blood or their stool is black as tar. In this situation you must see a doctor immediately. An emergent endoscopy must be done to determine the exact source of the bleed and then cauterize the bleeding area if it is actively bleeding.

2. If a person has very mild non-emergent symptoms of excess acid production, my first moderation approach is to make non-pharmacologic lifestyle changes.

    ○ This includes changing the time a person eats. Don't eat a short time prior to going to bed. Remember the highest acid production in the 24 hour time cycle is around midnight. You will also produce extra acid at that time in response to breaking down the food.

    ○ If a person has any acid reflux at all, laying down when going to bed can aggravate that reflux because it is simply a lot easier for the stomach acid to enter the esophagus in that position than if you are in a more sitting up position with your chest elevated. Try to elevate the head of the bed so that at night you can use gravity to keep acid from rolling back up from the stomach into the esophagus.

○ Be wary of overeating, which can produce excess acid production.

○ Try to eliminate or decrease food or drink that can increase a person's acid secretion. A main source for this is alcohol and caffeine. Caffeine is a huge culprit now with the presence of so many coffee shops that seem to be at every corner and all the caffeinated energy drinks that contain high levels of caffeine.

○ It is also important to look inward and determine if we are dealing with a lot of stress. If it has been severe, it can be associated with increased acid secretion. I try to always ask my patients who have the excess acid symptoms about their personal and occupational stressors. The saying that you have a "gut feeling" about something definitely has its origins in excess acid secretions related to stress. Doing relaxation techniques such as meditation, yoga, biofeedback, or talking to a counselor may help that excess acid secretion better than anything.

3. There are certain medications that can increase acid secretion. The most notable are the arthritis medications like the NSAIDS (non-steroidal anti-inflammatory drugs). Examples of NSAIDS are ibuprofen and naprosyn. They help in pain relief and lower inflammation; however, they can cause significant increase in acid secretion. If possible, I will try to get my patients who are

taking these drugs to decrease their usage and to switch to an herbal, such as ginger. Ginger has been shown to help arthritis pain and swelling without increasing acid secretion. The simple rule is if you are on a new medication and your stomach is now upset, the answer is usually pretty obvious. If it is a medication prescribed by your doctor, please contact your doctor first before stopping the medication unless the symptoms are a quite severe.

4. If a person has significant findings, such as a true ulcer, gastritis (inflammation of the lining of the stomach), or esophagitis, there is then no question that they should be placed on a medication. At the same time, lifestyle changes need to be instituted. I try to limit the time a person is on a PPI or H2 blocker to one to two months unless your gastroenterologist insists you stay on it longer because of an underlying condition such as Barrett's Esophagus. After one to two months I try to wean my patients off their PPI or H2 blocker. Many times by changing a person's lifestyle, and stopping acid-promoting medications, a person may be able to stop their PPI or H2 blocker. I generally start patients on H2 blockers first and then switch them to PPIs if the H2 blockers do not seem to be effective. If a person ends up on a PPI for one to two months, I then try to wean them off their PPI and switch them to an H2 blocker. After a month I will attempt to stop the H2 blocker. Not everyone can go off these meds, but staying on the lowest dose or amount may decrease the risk of some of the previously stated side effects.

12

The Opiate Addiction Crisis

Who is to blame? Should all opioid use end?

In our country today opioid overdose accounts for 63 percent of drug related deaths. In fact, the estimated number of drug deaths in 2016 topped the *total number* of soldiers killed in the Iraq and Vietnam wars. The Center for Disease Control estimates that 72,287 people died from drug overdoses in 2017, an increase of about 10 percent from the year before. A majority of the deaths—nearly 49,000—was caused by opioids. In 2017 Art Levine wrote a 2017 *Newsweek* opinion piece titled "Hard Truths About Psych Drugs: What I Learned, Eventually, from My Mother's Death in a Psych Ward" about his mother's accidental death from a fall after being over-medicated by sedatives and antipsychotic drugs during treatment at a well-respected hospital.

According to Levine, who authored the book *Mental Health, Inc.,* we are in the one of the worse epidemics of opiate addiction this country has ever seen. And we have certainly not learned from the past failures and malpractices of our physical and mental health systems that have contributed to this current crisis by overprescribing pain relief drugs and psychiatric medications.

Opiates in the Practice of Medicine:
The Prevalence of Opium Use in Earlier Times

Opiates that originally derived from the opium poppy have been used for physical and mental pain relief seemingly from the beginning of time. Archaeological evidence of its human use during rituals was found as long ago as the 5000 BCE during the Neolithic Age.[87] Sumerian clay tablets discovered at Nipper, south of Baghdad, record the first use of opium in Mesopotamia around 3000 BCE. The text describes the cultivation of the poppy plant and collection of poppy juice in the mornings. They named opium "Gil," the word for happiness.[88] The Assyrians also had a name for the poppy juice, and ancient Babylonian and Egyptian writings have many references to the use of opium preparations for pain relief.[89]

Much later in the eleventh century soldiers [90] returned from the Crusades with an addiction to opium. It was prevalent in Muslim societies from the fourteenth century onward. Turkey supplied the West with opiates long before it came to us from India and China.

In Europe in the 1500s, the highly addictive drug laudanum was created by combining a 10 percent solution of opium power in alcohol. It was widely used as a painkiller, cough suppressant, and sleeping aid as well as a recreational drug throughout the 1700s. By the 1800s, laudanum was the Victorians favorite medicine and readily available for purchase at grocers, pubs, and pharmacies. Many stories are told of the English Romantic poets and other British writers and artists who used it to enhance their feelings of euphoria and expand their creative powers, and who suffered illness and early tragic deaths from drug overdose. Coleridge composed his most famous poem "Kubla Khan" under the influence of laudanum and also suffered health and emotional problems from his addiction to opium throughout his life.

It should be noted that compared to the other chemicals used medicinally in the 1700 and 1800s, a solution containing opium was the physician's best alternative to prescribing arsenic, mercury, and other dangerous medicines. They successfully used opiates to treat major diseases like dysentery and respiratory illnesses as well as ordinary non-life threatening ailments.[91]

One reason opiate addiction became so widespread in the United States during the Gilded Age was the outcome of the Civil War.[92] Thousands of wounded and ill soldiers were treated with opium and morphine in field hospitals. When the survivors returned home to their heartbroken families and communities they had drug addiction to contend with along with their devastating losses. Studies have found that addiction was much worse in the South than elsewhere in the United States. Confederate soldiers and Southerners, especially white men and women, commonly sought solace from the destruction of their way of life by turning to opiates.[93]

We should rid ourselves of any notion that these were largely male addicts. Several official state surveys of Americans during the late 19th century revealed the majority of opiate addicts were female. One source of data reported that the highest rate of female addiction was in Albany where "fully four fifths" of opium-eaters are women."[94]

The Discoveries of Morphine and Codeine

In 1804 a German pharmacist was the first to isolate the active ingredient of morphine from the opium poppy plant. He named it *morphium* after the god Morpheus, the Greek god of dreams, because of the drug's sedative effect.[95]

In 1827 the Merck company, the world's oldest operating chemical pharmaceutical company founded in 1668 in Darmstadt,[96] Germany, began to market it commercially.

It became the most commonly prescribed drug for the relief of severe pain, and its other effects of feelings of detachment and euphoria make it one of the most popular and, unfortunately, highly addictive medications.[97]

About 70 percent of morphine is used today to make other opiates such as heroin, but morphine in itself continues to be a very valuable drug, the gold standard for the effective and safe treatment of acute and chronic pain for injuries and major diseases such as heart attacks and cancer. Morphine is on the World Health Organization's List of Essential Medicines.

In 1830 in France the chemical compound to make codeine was also "isolated" from the opium poppy plant. It was less powerful in its action as an analgesic than morphine, and as a medicine was prescribed primarily as a cough remedy. Many become addicted to these solutions of prescription-grade cough medicine, and because they are less-regulated than many other opiates and can be gotten quite easily, codeine is often considered more dangerous than morphine. It can be very harmful when mixed with large amounts of alcohol and soft drinks and can lead to abuse of other drugs like heroin, morphine, and oxycodone.[98]

Clint Lawson wrote in the *New York Times* in his article, "America's 150-Year Opiate Epidemic," that the last major opiate epidemic occurred between the 1870s and the 1920s, and our current epidemic began shortly after this.

Stories of drug addiction back then were not too dissimilar from the what we hear today. Physicians liberally prescribed morphine derivatives for all sorts of ailments, often by way of hypodermic needles, for everything from mental illness to toothaches and many other minor ailments. As terrible as it sounds, we must remember that the state of medical care at that time was abysmal at its best. We did not yet have antibiotics or any of the many lifesaving procedures we have now. With no significant therapies available, the medical world was happy to have at least one medication to help patients with their pain and suffering and to enable very ill people to breath, to relax, and to sleep peacefully.

As the number of uses for morphine and codeine increased, it was only a matter of time before the general public in America decided that the use of opiates could be justified beyond the physical therapeutic usages. This was the beginning of the world of addiction to opiates.

||||||||||||||||||||||||||||||||||||||||||||||||||||||||||||||||||||||||||||||||||||||||||||||||||||||||

THE OPIUM WARS

By 1830 the British public's dependence on opium was at its peak. In 1839 the British sent warships to the coast of China when China suddenly ordered a blockade and confiscated 1,210 tons of British opium grown in India and confined the foreign traders. China wanted to control trade agreements and the profits made by Western middle men, and was equally worried that in spite of their imperial prohibition of trading in opium, the lifting of restrictions for trading the drug would create an epidemic of opium addiction among their people. This incident was the beginning of the First Opium War (or the Anglo-Chinese War) that the Chinese regarded as unjust imperialist impositions. But China's military defeats forced them to open many ports to foreign traders that included Britain, the United States, Turkey, India, and Southeast Asia. Opium flooded into China and the use of opium filtered into all levels of society.*

||||||||||||||||||||||||||||||||||||||||||||||||||||||||||||||||||||||||||||||||||||||||||||||||||||||||

* from essay by Peter C. Perdue The first Opium War: The Anglo-Chinese War of 1839–1842 (MIT Visualizing Cultures)
https://ocw.mit.edu/ans7870/21f/21f.027/opium_wars_01/ow1_essay_01.pdf

The Development of Heroin and Oxycodone

Heroin, the first partially synthetic opioid, was manufactured in 1898 by Bayer. It was marketed as a nonaddictive substitute for morphine—even promoted as a product safe for children to use as a cough medicine.[99] But it turned out that heroin was twice as potent and more addictive than morphine.[100]

Likewise oxycodone, also a semi-synthetic opiate, was derived from an organic chemical Thebaine found in Persian and opium poppies that is similar to codeine. When Bayer introduced the drug to the market in 1916 it was promoted as a less addictive analgesic than morphine or heroin.[101]

Oxycodone was introduced to the United States in 1939, and in our century is now the active ingredient of OxyContin and many other commonly prescribed pain relief medications such as Percocet, Percodan, and Vicodin. These synthetic medicines all contain a small amount of oxycodone combined with other active ingredients like aspirin. Since oxycodone's chemical structure is similar to codeine, and it is almost as potent as morphine, it produces the same opiate effects as those drugs.[102]

There is a high risk of addiction and abuse of these pain killers that should be used when prescribed by a physician and under a doctor's care, but that are now often procured illegally and used on a long-term basis to achieve a euphoric mood. Many people who abuse these drugs start out taking them as prescription drugs for their physical pain. But their body develops a tolerance to it and they require higher and higher dosages to feel better and end up buying it illegally as they become increasingly in trouble both physically and mentally.

In the beginning of the 20th century the US government realized the severe effects of the epidemic of drug addiction and enacted several laws to prevent this. The United States Congress banned the use of opium in 1905 and passed the Pure Food and Drug Act of 1906 to require labelling the contents of all medicine. The Harrison

Anti-Narcotic Act of 1914 and the Heroin Act of 1924 followed. This helped to decrease the addiction rate but the problem never went away. Instead, it went underground and was considered to be a problem of the poor, the downtrodden who lived in the intercity.

Our Current Opiate Epidemic

Today we are again in the midst of a major epidemic of addictions. How did this happen? Could it have been prevented? Extreme choices once again put us in a place we shouldn't be. Instead of using good medical discretion, we went overboard in our use of opiates and opioids to treat pain.

Measuring Pain Relief: The 5th Vital Sign

The road to our present epidemic started in 1990 when Dr. Mitchell Max, who was the President of the American Pain Society, wrote a landmark editorial in the *Annals of Internal Medicine*. In his article he stated how there was no advancement in the treatment of pain over the previous twenty years.[103]

He thought that this failure was attributed to the following:

- Patients failed to let their medical care providers know they were in significant pain.
- Nurses did not have the ability to adjust dosage.
- Doctors were reluctant to use opiates.
- Pain was "invisible." Information about the patient's pain was not displayed in their medical chart
- Physicians were not held accountable for inadequate pain control.

Because of this observation, Dr. Max made the following recommendations:

- Make the patient's pain "visible."

- Give practitioners "bedside" tools to guide physicians and nurses to initiate and modify analgesic treatments.

- Assure patients a place in the "communications loop."

- Increase clinician accountability by developing "quality assurance guidelines," improving care systems, and assessing patient satisfaction.

- Facilitate innovation and exchange of ideas.

- Work with narcotics control authorities to encourage therapeutic opiate use.

The following year the American Pain Society introduced the following recommendations based on what Dr. Max had suggested:

- Hospital charts should clearly document the intensity of a patient's pain and the specific medications that were being used to treat the patients pain.

- A simple, valid measure of pain intensity should be selected by each unit

- Each clinical unit should identify values for pain intensity rating and pain relief rating that will elicit a review of the current pain therapy.

This resulted in 1999 having the California's legislature pass Assembly Bill 791, which added to the Health and Safety Code (HSC) that "Every health facility licensed pursuant to this chapter shall, as a condition of licensure, include pain as an item to be assessed at the same time as vital signs are taken. The pain assessment shall be noted in the patient's chart in a manner consistent with other vital signs." This was the beginning of the measurement of the 5th vital sign (the other four traditionally reported vital signs are a person's blood pressure, heart rate, respiratory rate, and temperature).

In 2000 after a three-year study, Dr. O'Leary the president of the Joint Commission, emphasized the need for organizations to do systematic assessments and use quantitative measures of pain (e.g., place pain on a ten-point scale). In addition to the standards themselves, the Joint Commission compiled a manual that brought all of the standards together into one place.[104]

The Joint Commission standards were hailed by pain management specialists and called "a rare and important opportunity for widespread and sustainable improvement on how pain is managed in the United States." A numeric pain scale became "mandatory" in the post-anesthesia care unit (PACU), and an "acceptable" pain score was required for discharge from the PACU.[105] The average consumption of opiates per patient increased from 40.4 mg (morphine equivalents) in 2000 to 46.6 mg in 2002, with the greatest increase in the PACU (6.5 mg to 10.5 mg).[106]

OxyContin Enters the World of Opioids

A further explosion of opioids production leading to our current epidemic occurred in 1995 with the approval of the prescription of the sustained-release opioid OxyContin. The Food and Drug Administration (FDA) approved labelling saying that iatrogenic addiction was "very rare" and that the delayed absorption of OxyContin reduced the abuse liability of the drug. These same claims were used in marketing campaigns to physicians and in more than forty national pain-management and speaker training conferences for which all expenses were paid. The FDA required removal of these unsubstantiated claims from OxyContin's labeling in 2001. However, the concept that iatrogenic addiction was rare and that long-acting opioids were less addictive had been greatly reinforced and widely repeated, and studies refuting these claims were not published until several years later. With this the number of prescriptions per million increase from 97 million in 1997 to 219 million in 2011.[107]

More specifics on this OxyContin story was that Purdue Pharma worked collaboratively with the VA on this drug. Purdue Pharma

gave $200,000 to the VA and promoted poorly done studies show-
ing that OxyContin rarely caused addiction.[108] The usage of opioids
skyrocketed in the VA with these poorly performed studies. When
the evidence about these poor and false studies about opiates were
made public, the VA swung completely in the other direction and
significantly cut off the dispensing of opioids. It was a disaster. When
60 percent of the veterans coming back from the Middle East were
diagnosed with chronic pain, many were placed on these long acting opiates like OxyContin because the "studies" said they were not
addicting.[109] When the VA received the information that the long-acting opiates actually were extremely addictive, they suddenly reversed
their recommendations on opiates use and decided to slash the frequency of their usage. As a result, the total amount of opioids prescribed by the VA since 2012 has dropped by over 50 percent.[110] This
caused severe panic among veterans. It would appear that it may be
one of the major factors that has led to the increasing number of sui-
cides of veterans.

The Physician's Role in Decisions About Opioid Use

All this conflicting information about analgesics occurred during
my time as a practicing physician. The information that we received
as physicians was very confusing. First of all, no doctor wants their
patient to suffer. That is why most of us went into medicine in the
first place. Our job is to treat the sick and rid people of their physical
and emotional suffering. As a physician my first job is to attempt to
cure an individual of their illness. If it isn't possible to cure the patient
of their disease, or they have some protracted illness that is taking a
long time to resolve, the last thing you want for any patient is to have
them suffering with pain.

I initially welcomed the hyper-vigilance of "keeping ahead of
the pain," as we used to say, and we believed we could accomplish

this. The first group we focused on were the hospital patients. These patients generally had acute illnesses, and as a physician I did not want them to suffer as I was treating their medical problems. When I first started using the 5th vital sign in the hospitals it seemed like the right move. I was told by the pain experts to get ahead of the pain by getting it under complete control rather than partially treating it. In addition, we were told that if we were more proactive with our treatment of pain, the patients were more relaxed, which ultimately led to their using less pain medication.

In the mix of this there was always the hospital's overriding fear about when they were going to be reviewed by the Joint Commission.* The hospitals were constantly internally evaluating themselves based on either how they did on the last review from the Joint Commission or whether they were ready and prepared for the next review by the Joint Commission. I remember the focus on this when making morning rounds at the hospital to see patients. A physician is commonly accompanied on each floor of the hospital by one of the floor staff nurses. Their responsibility was to care for the patients all the rest of the day, so they wanted to be sure they were following up on what the doctor ordered.

When all the hysteria about measuring the 5th vital sign and the responsibility to control the patients pain was at its peak in the

---

*The Joint Commission on Accreditation of Healthcare Organizations is a private, not for profit organization established in 1951 to evaluate health care organizations that voluntarily seek accreditation. The Joint Commission evaluates and accredits more than 16,000 health care organizations in the United States, including 4,400 hospitals, more than 3,900 home care entities, and over 7,000 other health care organizations that provide behavioral health care, laboratory, ambulatory care, and long-term care services. The Joint Commission also evaluates and accredits health plans and health care networks. It is governed by representatives from the American College of Physicians, the American College of Surgeons, the American Dental Association, the American Hospital Association, the American Medical Association, an at-large nursing representative, six public members, and the Joint Commission President. (https://www.jointcommission.org/)

early 2000s, the nurses constantly made me aware of where a patient was on the pain scale. This occurred even when a patient had an illness that typically was not associated with significant discomfort. As I made my rounds, the nurse would glowingly tell me what the patient's pain scale was and assure me that it was well documented so we need not worry about the Joint Commission docking their hospital floor during inspection. If the patient had an illness associated with pain, the physician was always the first to know if the patient's pain was not controlled. The nurses would often advise the doctors if we needed to change the type of pain medication or increase the strength.

I personally have seen the panic and fear in patients who become desperate when they need and want their opioids and can't get them. The only time in my medical career in which I was threatened and thought I was going to be killed was when I was attempting to wean down and possibly discontinue a couple's opiate usage. The husband was an ex-Marine who had an accident when he was in the service and permanently damaged his leg. He had a limp, was dependent on a cane, and suffered from chronic leg pain. When I saw him he was taking large amounts of opiates and constantly asking me to increase his dosage. His wife had severe, recurrent migraine headaches. She came to my office almost weekly for Demerol shots and her daily opiates. In those days there was no such thing as pain centers, so the primary care physicians were responsible for the total care and management of pain for their patients. I was very concerned about the amount of pain relievers I was prescribing for this couple. I felt I needed to find some way of decreasing their usage of opiates and to attempt to wean them off their medications.

I was one of the last doctors to still have evening office hours and had appointments with patients three evenings a week. I had been trying over the previous month to slowly decrease the amount of opiates this couple was taking. I was constantly receiving phone calls from the pharmacy requesting refills on their meds before their prescriptions were due to run out. The couple had made the last appointment of the evening to see me. When I had evening hours it usually was much quieter than during the day. This time they were the only patients who remained in my office.

When I walked into the couple's exam room and sat down I could tell they were both upset. When I asked them why they had come to see me, they said they wanted to talk about their medications. They asked if I was trying to decrease their medication amount and dosage. When I confirmed that I was attempting to do that, they wanted to know if instead they could have more medication than what I was prescribing. I told them I could not keep giving them such high dosages of opiate medication.

The ex-Marine did not respond to me but asked his wife to leave the room. As soon as she left, he stood up between me and the exit door and pulled a weapon out from behind him. It happened so quickly that all I saw was a long stick that I initially thought was a rifle. Then I realized it was not a gun but a type of Billy club.

He swung it at me as I dove behind the exam table. I screamed "911" as loud as I could from behind the table, hoping my nurse or receptionist would hear me. Fortunately they heard me, and both rushed to the exam room to see what was going on, and my nurse and receptionist ran to open the door. They both gasped and quickly shut the door again. Knowing that I am alive and survived the situation, the action of my loyal assistants gasping and closing the door was actually quite funny (only now can I laugh!). My patient swung the club at me again, and again missed me. I have never seen so much anger in a person's eyes, before or since. He then turned around, opened the door, and walked out of my office. His wife had been waiting in the car, and they drove away and never returned. Clearly, they were so addicted to their opiates nothing else in life mattered. I've never forgotten that evening and think of it every time I prescribe an opiate to a patient.

So what did all this policy of dispensing pain medications create? Just where we are today in another opiate crisis. I know there will always be abusers of medications, especially in the use of opiates. Anything that makes us feel better than our actual living conditions will always be in demand. It is our human nature to want to escape our physical and mental discomfort, to do something to elevate our moods. It is also our nature to find it almost impossible to have the will power to do this safely when we are so easily addicted to these chemicals. The medical establishment must take some of the responsibility for this.

Instead of taking a cautious and moderate approach to opiate use, our profession used poor judgment. We may have had good intentions, but we took a rash approach of excessively promoting opiates for pain relief and contributed to the disastrous result of addiction. The fear and anxiety over prescribing pain medications also led to overreactions of withholding drugs indiscriminately from patients who might have benefited greatly from our lessening their physical suffering.

WHAT IS THE MODERATION APPROACH TO THE USE OF OPIATES AND OPIOIDS?

1. First and foremost, if a person has severe acute pain, like a kidney stone, or if they are having severe postoperative pain, as long as a person is not allergic to an opiate, this is a definite indication for their use. Pain and suffering are not necessary. If, however, a person had a surgical procedure done and they were not in significant pain, it is then time to start decreasing and stopping their opiates.

2. Nighttime pain within the first few days after a surgery or a traumatic accident may mean a need to take an

opiate at night in order to sleep. Almost everyone with pain will have their pain amplified at night because of a lack of distractions from their environment. Poor sleep will also ultimately exacerbate pain. Therefore getting good sleep can improve a person's pain threshold. No one wants to be in pain. The last thing we want to do is eliminate pain meds at a time like this.

3. What is tricky is treating chronic pain. The first step in treating chronic pain is to first determine if there is any correctable cause for the pain. If this is found, the simple answer is to give relief by correcting the cause. An example of this is chronic hip pain as a result of severe degenerative arthritis. A patient may have tried physical therapy, non-steroidal medications like ibuprofen, or have intermittently been given steroids. These therapies may have helped for a while, but often there comes a point when these modalities are no longer successful. When this happens, a person starts to limit their activity, and with decreased physical activity, a person's risk of diseases increases. At this point many patients start requesting stronger and stronger pain meds to just get around and to be able to sleep at night. I see patients all the time who have severe painful arthritis when they come to Canyon Ranch. They often request opiates so they can exercise and "enjoy" their time at the ranch. This is when I often sit down with the patient and discuss with them the possibility of surgically obtaining a total hip. This procedure is so commonplace now, and the risk of complications under the hands of an excellent orthopedic surgeon is so low, that the best solution to their chronic pain is likely not the use of opiates but having a surgical replacement of the hip.

4. Unfortunately the answer to chronic pain is not often a simple surgical procedure. There are so many pain syndromes that have no cures. When this happens it is then up to the patient and their care provider to determine the best mode of therapies to deal with the pain. Most of us don't want to spend considerable time and effort on solutions to deal with chronic pain. We just want to take a pill and have it go away. This is where opiates have stepped in to give us that quick and easy answer. But opiates are rarely the best long-term answer. Beyond the problem of addiction, there are so many other consequences associated with chronic opiate use. People become tolerant to the dosage, so it is not unusual for a person to want and need more and stronger opiates to treat the chronic pain. Outside of the terrible addictive nature of these drugs, their effects often cause relationship issues. Most individuals become dulled from medications. They aren't as sharp and their communication skills go down, which causes difficulties in all their relationships, from the home to their work environment. There are a whole lot of safety issues they need to be aware of with the use of opiates that dull our senses and increase the risk of accidents. They must be very careful if they are living or working in an environment that needs excellent balance or operating a motorized vehicle or equipment that needs a person's full attention.

5. Maximize non-pharmacologic, non-surgical therapies for pain. This is a big list. Being a physician who is trained in integrative medicine, I have more options for a patient than the majority of other physicians. I can offer multiple alternative therapies in addition to traditional therapies

like physical therapy. There are modalities like acupuncture, neuromuscular therapy, and chiropractic therapy that have been shown to be helpful in many circumstances. I have one patient who was told she needed bilateral total knee replacement five years ago, but she returns to see me twice a year for acupuncture, and she still has not had the surgery. Mind-body medicine such as hypnosis can be effective for chronic pain. A patient of mine was on high-dose opiates, antidepressants, and neuroleptics (medications that were originally made for seizures and found to dull chronic pain) like gabapentin. He had severe chronic back pain and had three major back surgeries. Despite his reservations, I convinced him to see one of our behavioral therapists, Amy, for hypnosis. When he finished his session with the therapist he was crying. He said during the session it was the first time in five years he was without pain.

6. One final note: Until we find an effective pain reliever that is not an opiate (there are a few in the pipeline that may be available in the next five years), we are still going to need opiates for severe pain. We should view it not as a curse but as a temporary reprieve from severe unlivable pain.

13

Menopause

Is hormone replacement therapy the right path?

O nce again we are dealing with a classic dilemma of extremes of opinions as to what to do about prescribing hormones for perimenopausal and menopausal women. Because I work at Canyon Ranch, a large percentage of my patients are perimenopausal and menopausal. Even though most of these women see a gynecologist, I am often asked for my opinion on whether or not they should take hormone replacement

Women are often confused about what to do, and their friends often make them even more confused. The women that are having a lot of menopausal symptoms, are usually the ones who feel that every woman needs to be on some type of hormone replacement. Friends that sailed right through menopause and had little if any symptoms and never took hormone replacement, cannot believe any woman would even consider taking hormone replacement therapy.

I obviously did not go through menopause and am not swayed by a good or bad experience with menopause. For that reason I have no personal biases about whether or not a woman should take hormone replacement. I simply look at the medical scientific studies and consult with the women who are trying to make an informed decision.

I listen to their own personal history and ask about their family history of health matters related to menopause to help them make the best decisions for them.

If you are a woman who is nearing menopause or in the midst of menopause and is trying to make the decision about whether to take hormone replacement, the first thing you need to know is how the normal female physiology works. The first question that should be answered is: What actually is menopause? It is the time period when menstruation ceases because a woman runs out of eggs in their ovaries.

At puberty a female has an astonishing number of around 300,000 eggs remaining from the one million to two million eggs she was born with.[111] Each immature egg (ovite) is produced in a follicle, a fluid-filled sac that makes estrogen. Usually only one follicle in the ovary during each monthly cycle is stimulated to release a complete egg, the ovum, that then waits to be fertilized by a sperm in the fallopian tube.

When women run out of eggs and stops this process of ovulation, they also run out of estrogen production in the ovaries. This causes a major drop in the body's estrogen production, but it is important to note that after menopause there is still a small amount of estrogen produced outside of the ovaries from fats cells and in the brain by an enzyme called aromatase.

In addition, the other hormone that is normally produced during the second half of the menstrual cycle, progesterone, is no longer produced because it comes from the post ovulation follicle, which is called the corpus luteum. When you don't have any more eggs, you no longer have any follicles to make a corpus luteum. When the number of follicles decreases it is not unusual that intermittently no follicle will be stimulated to the point of ovulation. If this happens a woman's periods can become irregular. There are many different versions of this time. Some women will intermittently not be able to ovulate the few remaining follicles every month, and this causes periods to become irregular and "missed." Other women may suddenly not have any follicles left to stimulate, and their periods will stop right then, and they will never have another period. Each woman has an individual path to menopause. If you know when the onset of your mother's menopause occurred, it can give you clues as to what age you might go through your change. But there are no certain hereditary guidelines for this.

So what are the symptoms of menopause, and why do women want to consider hormone replacement therapy at this time? With the lack of estrogen, which is the result of no longer having any follicles to be stimulated to make estrogen, a number of physical and emotional symptoms can occur. When a woman's body recognizes that there is a lack of estrogen, the brain signals the pituitary gland to produce high levels of FSH (Follicle Stimulating Hormone) to try to stimulate any potentially remaining follicles in the ovaries. It is the high levels of FSH that cause vasodilation and the symptoms of uncomfortable hot flashes and night sweats, and the accompanying anxiety.

Other physical symptoms associated with lack of estrogen are vaginal dryness, which can cause painful intercourse, increased risk of urinary tract infections, loss of bone (which increases the risk for osteoporosis), dry skin, heart palpitations, joint pain, headaches, and the very frustrating experience of weight gain. Women may also have breast engorgement and pain, dizziness, poor sleep, and tingling sensations of their skin.

Psychological symptoms associated with low estrogen are poor memory, an inability to concentrate, a depressive mood, irritability, mood swings, lack of energy, and decreased libido.

If hormones can help prevent all these terrible problems, then why in the world wouldn't every woman want to take supplemental hormones? It's because of that awful disease, cancer. When I first started medical school, rarely did anyone even talk about menopause. One of the first times the subject was brought up to a wide public audience was on the TV show, *All in the Family*. In an episode called "Edith's Problem" aired in 1972, Edith Bunker, played by Jean Stapleton, displays unusual behavior of dramatic emotional swings and a tyrannical temper as she complains of hot flashes. Edith and the men are quite mystified about what is wrong with her, but Gloria, Edith and Archie's daughter, explains to Archie that he needs to be more sensitive to Edith while she's going through menopause.

Before then it was a hush-hush problem that menopausal women were just supposed to endure. What we did know at the time was that when a woman's estrogen level dropped, it often caused a loss of bone density called osteoporosis. This places a person at a higher risk for bone fractures. Some women were given estrogen if they had low bone density, especially if they already had bone fractures. At that time estrogen was one of the few things we could offer women who had osteoporosis.

There was a big problem with estrogen replacement. There was an increased risk of uterine cancer. This increased risk makes sense when you understand what happens in the uterus with a normal menstrual cycle. There are three phases:

1. The first is the proliferative phase: This stage is the first step in preparing the uterus for pregnancy. The follicle stimulating hormone goes to work to stimulates ovarian follicles. This results in an increased production of estrogen. The estrogen helps to thicken the membrane lining of the uterus called the endometrium in preparation for a fertilized egg and possible implantation of an embryo.

2. Secretory phase: Right after ovulation, the release of a matured egg from one of the follicles or sacs in the

ovaries that contain, the now empty follicle, called the corpus luteum, produces estrogen and the hormone called progesterone, which increases blood flow to the endometrium as it solidifies the lining, making the uterus a better environment for a fertilized egg. If the egg is not fertilized and the woman does not become pregnant, with the aging and collapse of the follicle the production of estrogen and progesterone declines.

3. Menstruation: With decreased production of estrogen and progesterone in the uterus and there has been no conception, the built-up tissues are not necessary, and endometrial lining of the uterus is sloughed off. This shedding normally takes three to five days. Then the whole process starts over again.

If a woman takes only estrogen during her hormone therapy, this continues to build up the lining of the uterus. This continued growth increases the risk of uterine cancer.[112]

When I was in medical school, studies revealed that if a woman is given both estrogen and progesterone their uterine cancer risk was significantly reduced compared to women only taking estrogen. So if a woman has a uterus and has significant menopausal symptoms, she should simply take estrogen plus progesterone, right? Well not so fast. What about breast cancer?

It has been found that estrogen plus progesterone may slightly increase the risk of breast cancer[113] more than taking estrogen alone. Therefore, if you are a woman that does not have a uterus you should take estrogen by itself. In this case you are still at a slightly higher risk for having breast cancer. This should not be too surprising since we now know through studies that woman with a longer exposure to estrogen are at a higher risk for breast cancer.[114]

The other major considerations in your decision-making on whether to use hormone replacement therapy is if you have a family history of breast or ovarian cancer and/or if you have mutations associated with breast or ovarian cancer on your own personal genes. A strong family history of breast or ovarian cancer would be a first degree relative, which is your mother, sister, or child. If there appears to be a family history of breast cancer, you may then consider genetic consultation. If you are a woman with genes that place you at a higher risk for breast and/or ovarian cancer then you should think long and hard about hormone replacement. The most serious and talked about are the BRCA 1 or BRCA 2 gene mutations. These are the most publicly known and have the greatest risk of developing breast and ovarian cancer. There are however several other genetic mutations that are called small effect genes which impart a higher risk for cancer than the general population but not nearly as high a risk as BRCA 1 or BRCA 2 mutations. These small effect genes should be pointed out after genetic testing is performed and then discussed with a genetic counselor.

WHAT IS THE MODERATION APPROACH TO HORMONE REPLACEMENT THERAPY?

1. If you are a woman that has little if any symptoms and there is a strong family history of breast cancer, or you have genetic mutations that increase your cancer risk, then I would discourage the use of hormone replacement therapy.

2. If you are a woman under the age of 60 who is having significant symptoms that are truly affecting your life and your relationships, and there is little if any family history of breast cancer, you can easily consider taking hormone replacement. If you don't have a uterus, take estrogen

only. If you do have a uterus you need to take an estrogen plus a progesterone.

3. The first two approaches are the easy ones to decide upon. Now the more complicated questions. If you are a woman with significant menopausal symptoms, but have a family history of breast cancer, what do you do? This is a very personal choice. Is it worth your slight increased risk of having breast cancer? I have heard many women say their life is so miserable that it is well worth the risk. So they should consider taking hormone replacement. However, they need to be vigilant about having their breasts checked both manually and by imaging. This should be followed closely by their physician. There are many variables. For example, do they have dense breasts, which slightly increases their breast cancer risk and makes it more difficult to diagnose a breast cancer.

4. Some do's and don'ts

    ○ Make up your mind about whether or not you are going to take hormone replacement therapy within the first year of menopause (going one year without having a period). If you wait too long to take estrogen, a sudden surge of estrogen again after a year may increase your cancer risk.

    ○ Take the lowest dosage of estrogen that controls your symptoms. Prolonged estrogen exposure increases the risk of cancer, and obviously the higher the dose of estrogen the more likely there is of further increasing the odds.

    ○ Consider using an estrogen patch or topical estrogen preparation. Unless you develop a significant rash from topical estrogen or a patch, always try that first. When you use a topical estrogen, the estrogen bypasses the liver and many of the significant side effects, such as blood clotting, is decreased.

○ If you do have a uterus and you need to take progesterone, unlike estrogen, it is best to take progesterone orally. Topical progesterone does not seem to have the same protective effect against uterine cancer as oral progesterone.

○ Over the age of sixty many of the medical risks associated with hormone replacement therapy start to increase and you need to have a long discussion with your doctor about continued usage of hormone replacement.

14

Sleep Aids

Which one would work for me? Are they safe?

Sleep is a major issue for all of us. Good sleep, which for most people means seven to nine hours of uninterrupted sleep, is very important for your health. Lousy sleep is associated with daytime drowsiness, increased blood pressure, increased appetite, increased inflammation, increased risk for cardiovascular disease risk, and increased anxiety and depression. And that is just a partial list! I am blessed to have a sleep specialist, Dr. Param Dedhia, right down the hall from me. I have learned so much about the importance of sleep from Dr. Dedhia. It is one aspect of our lives that we all like to talk about but never really understand. We do know that if we don't get enough, the next day almost all of us will be grouchy and sleepy.

One thing that goes without saying is that we would all like to get a good night's sleep. We just feel so much better when we do. There is nothing better than getting up in the morning and feeling well-rested. One of my personal rituals is to get up in the morning, go for a run, quickly shower and dress, and drive to Starbucks to grab a cup of coffee and sit down and do some writing for about an hour before heading off to work. As I sit at Starbucks writing, I watch the steady stream of morning coffee drinkers come through to get their morning

Joe to wake themselves up so they can begin their day. I see all types of people, but it doesn't take long to determine who slept well and who didn't. You can always tell who is going to struggle at the beginning of the day and who is likely to be fine. You can quickly tell which individuals you would want to be your coworkers in the morning and those that you wouldn't.

There are many different kinds of sleep disturbances. There is sleep apnea, which means a person quits breathing at night (not a good thing!). There is restless limb movement, which means a person is squirming or moving around at night and preventing deep sleep. There is the whole realm of snoring, which not only disrupts the sleep of the sleeper; it disrupts the sleep of everyone else in the house. Those are all disruptive, but the most common complaint I hear from my patients about sleep is having difficulties falling asleep. This is a form of insomnia. Although both genders have this problem, women have a more difficult time with this than men. I am commonly asked by my patients about the safety of sleep aids. They want to know if sleep aids are harmful to them. They want to know if it is worse not to get to sleep or take a sleep aid and be able to fall asleep. They ask me if there are some sleep aids that are safer than others. Whenever I give a lecture to a group, no matter what my topic may be, I am almost always asked about how I feel about sleep aids.

Are you a drug addict if you use a sleep aid to help you fall asleep? No! Should you use sleep aids indiscriminately because they are harmless? The answer is No! It is not an all or nothing matter. Let's look into this issue. At bedtime you should first go to bed at a reasonable time and turn the lights out. You should be able to fall asleep within twenty minutes. If you consistently don't fall asleep within an hour, this is abnormal. So if you are an individual that struggles to fall asleep, my suggestions are to first look at your nighttime rituals and try to determine if your sleep hygiene is maximized before any type of sleep aid should be suggested.

Good sleep hygiene consists of the following:

- Try to wind yourself down before getting into bed. Don't wind yourself up with an action-packed movie, doing work on complicated financial issues or doing extensive internet searches. Don't go to do a work-out at the gym late in the evening and then go directly home and try to fall asleep.

- Play soft (not hard-rock) music. Take a hot bath. Or do anything that is relaxing to turn down your mind, not rev it up.

- Consider meditating. Two really good phone apps for meditation are Headspace and Calm. Meditation helps quiet the mind and puts you in a much better space to relax and fall asleep.

Here are some additional sleep hygiene techniques:

- Sleep as long as necessary to feel rested (usually seven to eight hours for adults), and then get out of bed.

- Maintain a regular sleep schedule, particularly a regular wake-up time in the morning.

- Try not to force yourself to sleep.

- Avoid caffeinated beverages after lunch.

- Avoid alcohol near bedtime

- Avoid smoking or other nicotine intake, particularly during the evening.

- Adjust the bedroom environment as needed to decrease stimuli (for instance, reduce ambient light, turn off the television or radio)

- Avoid prolonged use of light-emitting screens (laptops, tablets, smartphones, and e-books) before bedtime.[115]

- If possible, try to resolve problems that you are worried about before your bedtime.

- Exercise regularly for at least twenty minutes, preferably more than four to five hours prior to your bedtime.[116]

- Avoid daytime naps, especially if they are longer than twenty to thirty minutes or occur late in the day

- If you have tried improving your sleep hygiene, but still have significant problems trying to fall asleep, at this point you may consider an aid to help you sleep. The first sleep aid that is most physiologic (characteristic of or appropriate to our body's normal functioning) is melatonin. In humans melatonin is made in the pineal gland in the brain. It is made from the amino acid tryptophan that makes serotonin that is then metabolized into melatonin. It has a circadian production rhythm (a biological activity based on a 24 hour cycle). It makes up to ten times more melatonin at night than during the day. The production increases at sunset and peaks between 11:00 pm and 3:00 a.m.[117] The melatonin stimulates multiple receptor sites throughout the body. The receptor sites are on the brain and other organ sites. As we get older our ability to fall asleep often becomes more difficult. A big reason this happens is that the amount of production of melatonin of a seventy-year-old is one quarter the production of a young adult.[118]

Regarding the choice to supplement melatonin, an important fact is that we can be desensitized to melatonin if we take excessive amounts.[119,120] This is relevant to the prolonged use of high melatonin doses to promote sleep, particularly among older adults with insomnia who might inadvertently purchase excessively large doses of the hormone. With this concern of high dosage of melatonin causing desensitization of the melatonin receptor sites over time, I now recommend lower doses of melatonin, in the amount of 0.3 to 0.5 mg in the evening.

The other major reason I will gravitate towards melatonin as my first choice is that the side effect profile is relatively low. It consists of occasional headaches, dizziness, some confusion, and occasionally fragmented sleep.[121]

One other very important chemical in over-the-counter sleep aid, that seems like it is in every over-the-counter sleep aid, is diphenhydramine, which is generic Benadryl. It is what is in all the PM meds—Tylenol PM, Advil PM, etc.—and in many of the old standby sleep aids like Sominex. Diphenhydramine is best known as a very sedating antihistamine. In the past I commonly had my patients use this medication to help them fall asleep. It has been quite effective for many of my patients over the years. But unfortunately, what we thought was a benign drug, may actually have side effects. The majority of the side effects of diphenhydramine are caused by the fact that in addition to its antihistamine effects, it has anticholinergic effects. Anticholinergics lower the level of the neurotransmitter acetylcholine in the brain. Acetylchoine is a chemical released by nerve cells that sends signals to other nerves and muscles. Physicians have prescribed the drug Aricept for years as a treatment for Alzheimer's because Aricept increases the availability of the neurotransmitter acetylcholine.

Since taking diphenhydramine has the exact opposite effect on the brain, there was a concern that long-term use of diphenhydramine may increase the risk of dementia. The longer an anticholinergic medication was used, the higher the risk was of having dementia, although it was felt that the effects of this drug was a reversible form of Alzheimer's dementia; however, that may not be the case. A study that was written up in *JAMA* in 2015 supported this concern because it showed an increased risk of actual nonreversible dementia.[122]

It must be noted here that another group of drugs commonly used for insomnia are the tricyclic antidepressants such as amitriptyline (generic Elavil). These drugs also have anticholinergic effects and were included in the study. Patients taking these drugs showed the same increased risk of Alzheimer dementia as the patients taking diphenhydramine.

An additional problem that can occur in older men with enlarged prostates is that the anticholinergic effects can result in urinary retention. I have seen this problem commonly over the years when older men take Benadryl (or tricyclics) for one of a various reasons, which includes allergy and cold symptoms or just trying to fall asleep. I have had many a call by desperate men who after taking a sleep aid to help them fall asleep suddenly couldn't urinate. It was not unusual to have to send them to the emergency room in the middle of the night to have a urinary catheterization.

I'd like to address the use of stronger medications to help one sleep. There have been many prescription sleep aids over the years. Opiates were used in the 1800s and part of the first half of the 20th century. There are very few situations in which opiates should even be considered as a sleep aid. One of the few cases of this is discussed in the chapter on opiates when patients are in acute pain. An example are patients who are dealing with immediate post-operative pain. I think you can prescribe an opiate to treat the acute pain, which then allows the person to fall asleep. However, if pain is not involved in the reason someone cannot fall asleep, no opiates should be prescribed for that person.

One of the most common drugs used at this time to help people fall asleep at night is zolpidem (generic for Ambien). It is not an opiate or a benzodiazepine. It works by enhancing the activity of the inhibitory neurotransmitter, γ-aminobutyric acid (GABA), via selective agonism at the benzodiazepine-1 (BZ_1) receptor. Zolpidem does not have anxiolytic, myorelaxant, or anticonvulsant properties like benzodiazepines because it does not stimulate the BZ_2 receptor, which has that effect. Zolpidem is a very effective quick-acting hypnotic, but it is far from a perfect drug.

Eszopiclone (generic Lunesta) is also a nonbenzodiazepine that is selective for stimulating a specific BZ_1 receptor and does not give the other benzodiazepine effects. Eszopiclone is used for those individuals that have a hard time staying asleep because it has a much longer half-life of six hours when compared to zolpidem which has a half-life of one to four hours.

The side effect profile follows that of the nonbenzodiazepines: One of the biggest issues is sleep-related activities. A partial list of activities shown to occur while a person is actually asleep includes sleep-driving, doing laundry, preparing and eating food, having sex, and making phone calls. The other concern for anyone taking the drug for longer than two weeks, is the potential of having withdrawal symptoms. The major problem that can occur with withdrawal is rebound insomnia. When this happens, the first response of most people is to go right back on the drug.

The other group of sleep aids are the actual benzodiazepines. They have the effect of being an anxiety relieving and muscle relaxing medication as well as an anticonvulsant. Because of their antianxiolytic, tranquilizing effect this group of sleep aid medications has a much higher abuse rate than occurs with the nonbenzodiazepines. I try to avoid this class if I can, but there are always exceptions to every case. Occasionally I will have a patient who can't fall asleep or stay asleep because they are very anxious and they have tried and failed on Zolpidem or Eszopiclone. At this point they are becoming more wired and dangerously frenzied every day because of lack of sleep. Sleep deprivation can be a serious medical issue that can cause multiple psychological and physical problems. The consequences of not sleeping at some point outweighs the potential ill effects from these drugs. At this point I may prescribe a benzodiazepine to relax them and help them to finally get to sleep. I instill in these patients the idea that this is definitely a short-term fix.

There are a select few patients I have had over the years that just cannot sleep without taking a nonbenzodiazepine or a benzodiazepine. It is with these few patients that one has to deal with the lesser of the two evils. It is always better to sleep than to have many nights of not sleeping normally, and in these situations of chronic insomnia I will continue to write them a prescription as long as they do not show unfortunate side effects.

A Non-Pharmacologic Approach to Treating Insomnia

I would be totally remiss if I didn't discuss one of the most successful newer non-pharmacologic treatments for insomnia. This therapy is called Cognitive Behavioral Therapy for Insomnia or CBT-I. What is so good about this therapy is that it has been found to be as effective and in some studies even more effective than medication for insomnia. Many sleep specialists feel it should be the first-line treatment for insomnia. An excellent article "Overview of the Treatment of Insomnia" is on the website Uptodate.com.

The behavioral components of CBT-I described in this article include the following:[123]

- Establishment of a stable bedtime and wake time seven days per week
- Reduction in time in bed to approximate the total hours of estimated sleep (sleep restriction)
- Encouragement to use the bed only for sleep and sex; try to sleep only when sleepy; and get out of bed if anxiety occurs while unable to sleep (stimulus control)
- Sleep hygiene, which includes avoidance of substances that interfere with sleep, avoidance of naps to maximize

sleep drive, and optimization of the comfort of the sleep environment

The cognitive approaches that CBT-I addresses are described as the following:

- Anxious and catastrophic thoughts that are associated with sleeplessness

- Inappropriate expectations about hours of sleep

- Misattributions regarding the effects of sleeplessness

- Relaxation through progressive muscle relaxation, mindfulness, and meditation

What could be better? Just change your behavior and you'll not have to take medication that has the potential for significant side effects and even addiction. So why isn't this widely used vs. taking medication? First of all, we live in a society where people want quick fixes and that can be accomplished by just taking a pill at night. Next, it takes time to learn this technique; the therapy takes 4 to 8 sessions to complete. Finally, you have to be able to find a cognitive behavioral therapist who has been trained in CBT-I. There still aren't a lot of therapists who are trained in this therapy. For most of my patients that have serious problems with chronic insomnia, (depending on whether I think it's a right choice for their personality) I recommend that they at least look into CBT-I and see if it is available by a therapist in their community.

TAKING A MODERATE APPROACH TO SLEEP AIDS

1. Use good sleep hygiene nightly to improve sleep. (See lists at the beginning of this chapter.)

2. If you are unsuccessful with falling asleep in spite of following the normal rules of good sleep hygiene, you can

consider taking the supplement melatonin. But do not use a high dosage of melatonin because of the concern about becoming desensitized to it.

3. You can use over-the-counter diphenhydramine (Benadryl) intermittently, but it should not be used on a regular basis, especially because of recent study indicating that chronic use of this medication may cause long-term dementia.

4. Do not use opiates to help you fall asleep except in a rare situation when acute pain needs to be relieved to help you fall or stay sleep.

5. Stronger sleep aids can be considered by your doctor whenever a person has a pattern of being incapable of sleeping. The first medication in this list is zolpidem that is designed to be a quick-acting means of falling asleep. The drug eszopiclone can be used if a medication is needed to help you stay asleep. The last choice of medications that can be prescribed are the class of benzodiazepines if you can't fall asleep and you have high anxiety about it.

6. Remember that it is better to get some sleep from an artificially induced sleep aid than sleeping very little or not sleeping at all.

7. Finally, for those individuals that have chronic insomnia and especially those that are opposed to the usage of medications, I highly recommend looking into finding a cognitive behavioral therapist who is trained in CBT-I. In the short run it can be difficult and time consuming, but in the long run it may be the best thing you can do to treat your insomnia.

Environmental Toxins

15

The Contaminants Around Us

Which are the most dangerous?

Environmental toxins are becoming a bigger and bigger problem every year. The population of the earth continues to grow, and therefore there are more toxic wastes on this planet. The *Blade Runner* sequel gives a gruesome vision of where we are potentially headed if we don't do something. These toxins are causing many health issues.

Health care costs are going through the roof because of the many of illnesses and disorders that occur as a result of these environmental toxins. The estimated annual costs of pediatric care from the morbidities and mortalities associated with health issues directly related to environmental toxins that cause lead poisoning, asthma, cancer, and developmental disabilities is between $48.8–64.8 billion. This sum amounts to 2.8 percent of total US health care costs. This particular study looked only at these four areas of illnesses in children.[124] The total costs of health issues from toxins in our environment is much greater than this.

Air Pollution

With all the smog and the worsening air quality, more people are now developing respiratory problems such as asthma and recurrent bronchitis. We are all familiar with the primary air pollution and "ambient air quality criteria" or standards of our air measured by concentrations of pollutants that occur in or outdoor air. This is largely caused by fossil fuel emissions from cars, trucks, and buses that release carbon monoxide, nitrogen oxides, and other pollutants directly into our atmosphere. Secondary pollutions result from the chemical reactions among these elements in our atmosphere that can pose health problems throughout our lives. We are also exposed to other dangerous chemicals and gases at our work and in our homes.

Asthma is a well-known problem that can be caused by or exacerbated by environmental toxins, especially at work. It is usually caused by specific workplace sensitizers or irritants. Studies estimate that about 16 percent of all cases of adult-onset asthma are caused by occupational exposures.[125] Work-exacerbated asthma, which is the worsening of asthma due to the nature of our work, is common and estimated to have a median prevalence of 21.5 percent among asthmatic adults.[126]

This was seen with both outside air pollutants, work environments, and home environmental exposures. Exposure to the body parts and droppings of dust mites and cockroaches cause allergic reactions when they enter our air. This has been shown to contribute to an increase in both adult and childhood asthma and to mortality from this severe illness.

Air pollution has also been linked to increased rates of cardiovascular disease.[127,128] In fact, recent studies indicate that the greatest health threat from air pollution is cardiovascular disease caused by breathing dangerous small particles (particulate matters) that pass from our lungs into our blood stream.[129] The mechanism of the higher rates of cardiovascular disease may be related to the increased risk of developing high blood pressure that is noted in individuals exposed to air pollution.

Ambient air pollution causing exposure to particulate matters is also responsible for a considerable number of deaths from lung cancer and chronic obstructive pulmonary disease.[130]

Toxins in Our Soil and Water

Another major concern about environmental toxins is increased disease and cancer risk from toxins in our soil and water. This can be seen clearly in the obvious dangers of living next to a toxic waste dump (think Erin Brockovich). Every-day living requires being vigilant about the water we drink.

Destruction of Our Ozone

Other environmental agents that have been shown to cause disease indirectly are the chlorofluorocarbon gases. These are the kinds of gases used in refrigerators and spray cans that were destroying our ozone and are being phased out because of the famous Montreal Protocol, an international treaty enacted in 1989 to regenerate our ozone layer.[131] Because of the loss of much of this protective layer of the atmosphere there is an increase in ultraviolet radiation which leads to an increase in skin cancers, particularly melanoma.

Radon Contamination

This is the odorless tasteless radioactive gas that is produced from decaying uranium. It is found in the soil and rocks. High levels are seen in caves and mines. It is also found in water treatment facilities. It can be found in the basements of residential homes, especially if there are a lot of cracks in the foundation. The only way to determine if you have it in your home, especially the basement, is to test for it. The amount in the air is generally quite low. Another area of concern in radon contaminants is deep-well drinking water. The good news is that radon generally is quickly released as soon as it is exposed to the air.

The biggest concern of radon exposure is the increased risk of lung cancer. It is the second leading cause of lung cancer. Smoking, of course, is still the number one cause. A person generally needs a long exposure to radon to end up developing lung cancer by itself. However, the combination of radon exposure and being a smoker or recent ex-smoker significantly increases the risk of lung cancer.[132]

Contamination of Our Foods

In our time, the toxins in foods we eat are of great concern, and are especially problematic for those who are not eating organic produce. Farmers who are trying to get the best yield from their fields and don't want their crops to be eaten by insects found out that spraying their crops with fertilizers and insecticides enabled them to finally turn a profit in a very difficult profession. But what did all these chemicals on the plants do to the consumer?

Here are some unfortunate potential health problems that occur because of this. One of the diseases that has been looked at extensively is Parkinson's. This is a disease in which an individual has a decreased production of dopamine in the brain. It has long been thought that one of the causes of this is related to the usage of pesticides. There has been several studies that have shown that correlation.[133,134] Other diseases have also shown linkage to pesticides. One of the newer studies has shown a link to diabetes.[135]

The effects of pesticides are generally much worse for children than adults. A study done on children was performed in a country with one of the highest usages of pesticides, China. This study showed actual pesticide poisoning in children. It was done in the Zhejiang province of China. During the study period, totally 2,952 children were poisoned by pesticides. There were 66 deaths, resulting in a fatality rate of 2.24 percent.[136]

My patients frequently ask me if all foods are alike when it comes to pesticides. The answer is no. There are certain foods that have more exposure to pesticides than others. The Environmental Working Group measures levels of pesticides in foods. They have been putting out a list of foods since 2004 called the "Dirty Dozen." These are the fruits and vegetables known to have the highest pesticide contamination. This information was obtained from the United States Department of Agriculture (USDA). The Environmental Working group analyzed USDA pesticide residue data and found that almost 70 percent of nonorganic produce sampled tested positive for pesticide contamination! Below are the "Dirty Dozen" for 2018. The 2018 list included a 13th item because EWG found that hot peppers were contaminated with dangerous pesticides, and they suggest that organic ones should be bought:

1. Strawberries
2. Spinach
3. Nectarines
4. Apples
5. Grapes
6. Peaches
7. Cherries
8. Pears
9. Tomatoes
10. Celery
11. Potatoes
12. Sweet bell peppers
13. Hot peppers*

---

*A 13th item of hot peppers added in the 2018 list of the Dirty Dozen because of high levels of pesticides found.

The number one food on the list is strawberries because the USDA found that one third of all conventional, or nonorganic, strawberry samples contained ten or more pesticides. Spinach was the second on that list. It contained pesticide residues in 97 percent of nonorganic samples.

Of course one would like to know if there are fruits and vegetables that have lower contents of pesticides. Once again let's look at the Environmental Working Group for answers. The "Clean Fifteen" below are the recommendations for their 2018 list:

1. Avocados

2. Sweet corn

3. Pineapples

4. Cabbages

5. Onions

6. Sweet peas (frozen)

7. Papayas

8. Asparagus

9. Mangoes

10. Eggplants

11. Honeydew melons

12. Kiwis

13. Cantaloupes

14. Cauliflower

15. Broccoli

Mercury

If we are talking about toxicities and food, we need to talk about fish and mercury toxicity. The predominant source of organic mercury toxicity is contaminated fish. Certain types of marine fish (such as shark, swordfish, and tuna) and certain fish taken from polluted fresh waters (such as pike, walleye, and bass) may contain high concentrations of mercury, almost completely in the form of methyl mercury that can be dangerous to us. Other potential sources for exposure to organic mercury are wood preservation and outdoor painting. Excessive organic mercury consumption may present with subtle neurocognitive effects such as mild deficits in fine motor skills, verbal memory, and attention. But the effects of methyl mercury in children who were exposed as fetuses may be more severe.[137]

A MODERATION APPROACH TO ENVIRONMENTAL TOXINS

1. Beware that there are many environmental toxins that have the potential for causing disease. A very short list of the more harmful groups of toxins, and certainly far from the complete list, are radon, methyl mercury, and many of the chemicals causing air pollution.

2. I recommend that you go to the Environmental Protection Agency (epa.gov) site where it will inform you whether you are living in a high radon region. If you are, they tell you how to obtain a radon kit to test the levels where you live.

3. Unless you have chosen to be a vegetarian, you don't have to eliminate fish from your diet, which is a good source of low-fat protein and a good source of essential minerals and vitamin D and B2, and omega-3 fatty acids. Just be smart and well-informed about your selection of what kind of fish you eat. Try to stay away from predatory fish

like tuna, swordfish, and shark and fish living in areas of polluted fresh waters like bass, walleye, and pike. For more extensive lists of which fish are recommended to eat, go to the Monterey Aquarium website.

4. Wash your food carefully before you eat it. Many pesticides can be decreased by simple cleaning.

5. Whenever possible, try to eat organic foods. This will decrease the potential pesticides and toxins you can be exposed to in your food. If you occasionally eat some food that is nonorganic, the world will not end. We do have a very good detoxification system built into our bodies to deal with the occasional toxins that slip into our system when not always eating organic foods claimed to be free of pesticides.

6. Try to stay away from the "Dirty Dozen" as much as possible, and when you do eat fruits and vegetables, try to make it the "Clean 15."

16

Avoiding Toxins

Vaccination controversy: Whose advice do we follow?

There is no question environmental toxins are ever increasing on our planet. I am concerned about my daughter's future health and the health of generations to come. We must take action now to protect the next generations from environmental disease risks.

With that said, haven't we sometimes gone too far? One area in which this seems to be the case is in the controversy about vaccines that began with false accusations that vaccines cause multiple health issues.

One of the most commonly used vaccines for childhood, the MMR (measles, mumps and rubella) vaccine, contains the preservative thimerosal. It's added in small "trace amounts" to prevent formation of mold and bacteria in the multi-vial dosages distributed around the world during epidemics of these diseases. Thimerosal contains an organic mercury called ethyl mercury that is cleared from the body quickly, unlike methyl mercury that builds up in the human body and becomes a contaminant. In fact, thimerosal has been used in vaccines since the 1930s, and studies have indicated that is very safe when used in vaccines, although a very small percentage of people can be allergic to it.

Because of the public outcry about this, in 2001 thimerosal was reduced or removed from all recommended vaccines for children aged six years old and younger that are manufactured for the United States market. Multi-dose vials of flu shots for older children and adults contain influenza thimerosal, but single-dose vials for the vaccine that do not contain thimerosal are also available to older children, adolescents, and adults.[138,139]

With all the potential toxic effects of methyl mercury that I have discussed, it is perhaps understandable how a longstanding fear could emerge and grow among certain practitioners and lay public about the potential of toxic effects from vaccines, especially those containing thimerosal.

There have been no studies to support claims that it is harmful to the body and was well-known in the scientific community that thimerosal is a compound that breaks down into the form of ethyl mercury that our bodies are able to remove. This is a very different situation from what happens in our bodies with ingestion methyl mercury, the kind of toxin found in contaminated fish. Methyl mercury is hard for our bodies to filter out and can "bioaccumulate."[140] But the public as well as some members of the medical profession refused to be reassured about these scientific facts about mercury and fell prey to what seems to be unwarranted terror about vaccinations.

Thus in the 1990s, when integrative medicine had its beginnings and naturopathic medicine was on the rise, there was a major concern that vaccines, especially the MMR, were the source of many neurological diseases.

Since I was part of the original group of physicians involved in integrative medicine, I heard this concern vehemently expressed, and for many years these fears overwhelmed the public's ability to appreciate this great advance in medicine to extinguish deadly diseases that threatened their own children and humanity at large. I felt like I was in the minority of integrative medicine trained doctors who thought that vaccines were one of the most important scientific discoveries in the last three hundred years of medicine. This was a big deal in my practice because as a family physician I saw a lot of pediatric patients. When parents brought their children in to see me, I would hear their concerns about their various medical issues, and invariably they would ask questions about vaccines for their kids and themselves.

At the same time this was happening, there was an increased public awareness of autism. More and more people were talking in the public about the autistic spectrum. There were movies released with actors portraying autistics, including Dustin Hoffman's great portrayal of Raymond in the 1988 film *Rain Man*, which won Best Picture at the Academy Awards. Later TV shows had actors who portrayed high functioning people with Asperger's Syndrome, as in *Boston Legal*. Because more and more people were talking about autism, there was a public opinion that the disease was increasing in numbers. Some of that was true. The numbers increased slightly.

Then along came an article in 1998 in the famous peer-reviewed medical journal, *The Lancet*, about a study that describing an association between the vaccine MMR and autism.[141] This study was based on only twelve children as the subjects! The parents claimed that eight out of twelve of the previously normal children displayed behavioral symptoms within the spectrum of autism as well as symptoms of gastrointestinal disease within two weeks of receiving MMR vaccinations.

This study by Dr. Wakefield took the world by storm. It seemed as if many of the practitioners in the holistic medicine, integrative medicine, and naturopathic medicine world felt validated by this tiny study. These alternative-thinking practitioners felt these vaccines were causing harm. I was surrounded by these "free thinkers" who thought my ideas of vaccines were archaic, and if I continued to vaccinate my patients, I was responsible for being a part of the autism "epidemic." I remember well my consternation. I could not understand how a serious medical professional could toss out years of the findings of clinical work and academic research and base their opinion on one paper of a study with only twelve participants. It was that old adage that you only believe what you want to believe. This study caused so much uproar among parents that many were persuaded that all vaccines were causing toxic effects, and they began refusing to give any vaccines to their children.

A year after *The Lancet* published this article another study came out in which there were several hundred participants. It showed there was no causal relationship between the MMR vaccine and autism.[142] Years later, it was reported that Wakefield had received funding for his research and had personally received large sums of money from UK lawyers preparing a lawsuit against pharmaceutical companies that manufactured the MMR vaccine and had never informed anyone of his conflict of interest. In 2004 *The Lancet* formally announced the retraction of their interpretations of Wakefield's findings and ten of Wakefield's twelve co-authors of the paper later published their retractions.[143]

It is important to note that in 1999 the CDC and the American Academy of pediatrics requested as a precautionary move to have the pharmaceutical companies produce vaccines without thimerosal. The thimerosal was then slowly phased out of all the vaccines except for influenza. Despite this, the rate of autism has continued to rise.[144] Many articles since then have been published showing no correlation of autism and vaccines.

Unfortunately it wasn't until 2010, despite all the peer-reviewed articles that were out disputing Wakefield's findings, and long after Dr. Wakefield had been barred from practicing medicine in the United Kingdom where he lived and had worked, that the disputed original article was totally retracted from *The Lancet*.

But the damage had been done. Still to this day, I will get patients who will not allow their child to be vaccinated out of fear that their child will become autistic. This has been difficult for me to comprehend simply as a person, not as a doctor, since I personally had a severe case of each of the three prevalent childhood diseases the MMR vaccine was developed to prevent. I remember having the measles with a 103 degree temperature, covered head to toe with an extremely painful pruritic rash, and feeling like I was going to die. I still wear the scars on my face from a severe case of chickenpox, and, finally, I am so happy I was able to father a child, after having a severe case of the mumps. With each disease I had very serious and potentially life-threatening complications that fortunately I was able to recover from.

Even though we know there are serious toxins in the environment, there are many people that will take their fears and concerns about this to the extreme. They may avoid eating all fish because of their fear of mercury poisoning. They will drive for miles to buy all organic foods at high prices they cannot afford. They will go only to certain organic farmer's markets for seemingly irrational reasons and refuse to consume categories of food because they rely on unregulated supplements instead. They may move to inconvenient locations far from a city and their job to stay away from air pollution. They are so worried about the effects of vaccines they will not allow themselves or their children to have any vaccines. This can become costly, time-wasting, exhausting, and unfortunately could be outing themselves at risking a serious health problem.

A MODERATION APPROACH TO TAKING VACCINES

1. Please consider a policy of taking vaccines that are recommended by your doctor. Serious diseases can be prevented by these shots. Yes, there will always be that very rare individual, like literally one in a million, that may have a severe reaction to a vaccine. But this is by far the

exception, and if these diseases are not prevented by a community's "herd immunity" created by the vaccine's protection of a large number of the population, this will cause widespread and life-threatening illnesses. If your child had what was possibly a reaction to a vaccine, please discuss it with your doctor. More often than not, it will be explained that it did not seem to be a truly allergic reaction. However, If your doctor feels the reaction you or your child had after being given a vaccine was a vaccine reaction, then certainly that particular vaccine should never be given again to your child or to you.

2. Ask your doctor about good sources of articles or books about the medical issues that concern you so that you are up-to-date on these subjects and can make the best medical decisions for yourself and your family.

Epilogue

Taking extreme measures are generally unnecessary to be healthy or to attain the goal of improving your health. In some cases extreme behavior can actually be deleterious to your health. A reasonable approach to an exercise program should be a good workout to decrease the risk for chronic diseases, but at the same time does not consume us. Excessive exercise on the other hand has the potential of actually harming our bodies.

Following a strict and limited diet can be frustrating to maintain—and ultimately may not be healthy for us. A more moderate approach of eating more carefully and well can be healthy and also help with weight loss, if that is your objective.

Be aware of all the potential side effects of any long-term medication that may be prescribed by your doctor, whether it is by prescription or over-the-counter. Many times the potential side effects of using it for a long time are worse than the problem it is supposed to be treating. In addition, ask your physician if you are likely to need to stay on that prescribed medication indefinitely.

Most of the suggestions and discussions offered in this book emerge from basic common sense. Running to the point of complete exhaustion, eating food that tastes terrible to us because it's supposed to be healthy, and regularly taking medications that make us feel worse instead of better, are actions on the verge of insanity if we continue doing these things. A simple and easy rule of thumb is that if something doesn't seem logical, please question the validity of your recommended course by getting a second or third opinion before continuing down that path.

Just as I have been expressing what I have learned about the importance of avoiding extremes, I do not recommend that you only do those things that are simple and easy. Maintaining a healthy lifestyle does take a little discipline, or even quite a bit of work. Getting up at 5:30 in the morning to run several days a week isn't the easiest or most exciting thing to do. Staying away from those delicious pastries at the local bakery or having a big bowl of ice cream right before bedtime is very tempting, but must be resisted once we understand that this will in no way benefit our goal to improve our health.

At the same time, as you slowly make healthy choices and continue to push yourself towards healthier ways, you will get to a point where pushing yourself any further could negatively affect some very important moments in your lives—the moments when you occasionally have an ice cream cone with your child or times when you forgo your demanding exercise routine on a Saturday and limit your run to 45 minutes in order to spend the rest of an enjoyable morning with family and friends. This moderate approach will help you to balance your experiences and will ultimately bring you a healthier and happier life.

Notes

1. *J Cardiovasc Echography.* 2015 Oct-Dec; 25(4): 97–102. "Right Ventricular Changes in Highly Trained Athletes: Between Physiology and Pathophysiology" by Antonello D'Andrea, Alberto Morello, Agostino Mattera Iacono, Raffaella Scarafile, Rosangela Cocchia, Lucia Riegler, Enrica Pezzullo, Enrica Golia, Eduardo Bossone,1 Raffaele Calabrò, and Maria Giovanna Russ.

2. Susan A. Hall, et al., "Sexual Activity, Erectile Dysfunction, and Incidence Cardiovascular Events," *American Journal of Cardiology* 105:2 (2010): 192–197.

3. *Biol Sport.* 2016 Sep;33(3):215-21. doi: 10.5604/20831862.1201810. Epub 2016 May 1. "Temporal Associations Between Individual Changes in Hormones, Training Motivation and Physical Performance in Elite and Non-Elite Trained Men." Crewther, B.T., Carruthers, J., Kilduff, L.P., Sanctuary, C.E., Cook CJ5.

4. *Medicine and Science in Sports and Exercise,* 2017 Feb 13. "Endurance Exercise Training and Male Sexual Libido." Hackney, A.C., Lane, A.R., Register-Mihalik, J., O'Leary, C.B.

5. "The Growth and Development of Vegan Children." Sanders, T.A., Manning, J. *J Hum Nutr Diet.* 1992; 5:11.

6. "Size, Obesity, and Leanness in Vegetarian Preschool Children." Dwyer, J.T., Andrew, E.M., Valadian, I., Reed, R.B. *J Am Diet Assoc.* 1980;77(4):434.

7. "Gut Microbe-Generated Trimethylamine *N*-Oxide From Dietary Choline Is Prothrombotic in Subjects." Weifei Zhu, Zeneng Wang, W. H. Wilson Tang, Stanley L. Hazen. Circulation. 2017;135:1671-1673. Originally published April 24, 2017.

8. https://en.wikipedia.org/wiki/History_of_USDA_nutrition_guides

9. Scientific American.com. https://www.scientificamerican.com/article/rebuilding-the-food-pyramid/.

10. Healthcare (Basel). 2017 Jun; 5(2): 29. Published online 2017 June 21. doi: 10.3390/healthcare5020029 PMCID: PMC5492032PMID: 28635680 "Saturated Fatty Acids and Cardiovascular Disease: Replacements for Saturated Fat to Reduce Cardiovascular Risk." Michelle A. Briggs, Kristina S. Petersen, and Penny M. Kris-Etherton.·

11. "Cow's Milk Protein Allergy and Intolerance in Infancy: Some Clinical, Epidemiological and Immunological Aspects." Høst A. *Pediatr Allergy Immunol.* 1994;5(5 Suppl):1.

12. "Cow's Milk Allergy in Infancy." Heine, R.G., Elsayed, S., Hosking, C.S., Hill, D.J. *Curr Opin Allergy Clin Immunol.* 2002;2(3):217.

13. *J Hist Med Allied Sci* (2008) 63 (2): 139-177. DOI: https://doi.org/10.1093/jhmas/jrn001. 23 February 2008.

14. General background can be found in Hillel Schwartz, *Never Satisfied: A Cultural History of Diets, Fantasies, and Fat* (1986; New York: Anchor, 1990); Peter Stearns, *Fat History: Bodies and Beauty in the Modern West* (New York: New York University Press, 1997); Harvey Levenstein, *Paradox of Plenty: A Social History of Eating in Modern America* (1993; Berkeley: University of California Press, 2003). For the reducing diet habits of college women, see Margaret A. Lowe, *Looking Good: College Women and Body Image, 1875–1930* (Baltimore, MD: Johns Hopkins University Press, 2003).

15. https://www.nytimes.com/2004/11/23/obituaries/dr-ancel-keys-100-promoter-of-mediterranean-diet-dies.html.

16. https://www.sevencountriesstudy.com/about-the-study/history/.

17. Henry Blackburn, MD. "On the Trail of Heart Attacks in Seven Countries," University of Minnesota School of Public Health. https://sph.umn.edu/site/docs/epi/SPH%20Seven%20Countries%20Study.pdf Accessed 1.12.2019.

18. *Am J Med.* 2015 Mar; 128(3): 229–238. "The Mediterranean Diet, its Components, and Cardiovascular Disease." R. Jay Widmer, MD/PhD, Andreas J. Flammer, MD, Lilach O. Lerman, MD/PhD, and Amir Lerman, MD.

19. *Drug News Perspect.* 2008 Dec;21(10):552-61. "Fatty Acid Facts, Part III: Cardiovascular Disease, Or, A Fish Diet Is Not Fishy." Pauwels EK1, Kostkiewicz M.

20. "Effect of Early Introduction of Formula vs Fat-Free Parenteral Nutrition on Essential Fatty Acid Status of Preterm Infants." Foote KD, MacKinnon MJ, Innis SM. Am J Clin *Nutr.* 1991;54(1):93.

21. *Diabetes.* 2005 Jul;54(7):1926-33. "A High-Fat Diet Coordinately Downregulates Genes Required for Mitochondrial Oxidative

Phosphorylation in Skeletal Muscle." Sparks, L.M., Xie, H., Koza, R.A., Mynatt, R., Hulver, M.W., Bray, G.A., Smith, S.R.

22. Anderson, A.S., Haynie, K.R., McMillan. R.P., et al. "Early Skeletal Muscle Adaptations to Short-Term High Fat Diet in Humans Before Changes in Insulin Sensitivity." *Obesity*.2015;23:720-24.

23. *Front Endocrinol* (Lausanne). 2014; 5: 161. Published online 2014 Oct 9. "Insulin in the Brain: Its Pathophysiological Implications for States Related with Central Insulin Resistance, Type 2 Diabetes and Alzheimer's Disease." Enrique Blázquez, Esther Velázquez, Verónica Hurtado-Carneiro, and Juan Miguel Ruiz-Albusac.

24. "Effect of Low-Fat vs Low-Carbohydrate Diet on 12-Month Weight Loss in Overweight Adults and the Association with Genotype Pattern or Insulin Secretion." The DIETFITS Randomized Clinical Trial. Christopher D. Gardner, PhD; John F. Trepanowski, PhD; Liana C. Del Gobbo, PhD; et al. Michelle E. Hauser, MD; Joseph Rigdon, PhD; John P. A. Ioannidis, MD, DSc; Manisha Desai, PhD; Abby C. King, PhD. *JAMA*. 2018;319(7):667-679.

25. "Trends in Alternative Medicine Use in the United States, 1990-1997 Results of a Follow-up National Survey." David M. Eisenberg, MD; Roger B. Davis, ScD; Susan L. Ettner, PhD; et al. Scott Appel, MS; Sonja Wilkey; Maria Van Rompay; Ronald C. Kessler, PhD. *JAMA*. 1998;280(18):1569-1575.

26. *Am J Clin Nutr* January 2007. vol. 85 no. 1 265S-268S. "Multivitamin/Mineral Supplements and Prevention of Chronic Disease: Executive Summary 1,2,3." Han-Yao Huang, Benjamin Caballero, Stephanie Chang, Anthony J. Alberg, Richard D., Semba, Christine Schneyer, Renee F. Wilson, Ting-Yuan Cheng, Gregory Prokopowicz, George J. Barnes II, Jason Vassy, and Eric B. Bass.

27. https://www.healthline.com/nutrition/vitamin-a-deficiency-symptoms#section9

28. https://www.ncbi.nlm.nih.gov/pubmed/21457433/Liver Int. 2011 May;31(5):595-605. Jan 11. "Review of Liver Injury Associated with Dietary Supplements." Stickel, F., Kessebohm, K., Weimann, R., Seitz, H.K.

29. "Vitamin A Intake and the Risk of Hip Fracture in Postmenopausal Women," The Iowa Women's Health Study. L.S. Lim, L.J. Harnack, D. Lazovich, A.R. Folsom. Osteoporos Int. Author manuscript; available in PMC 2007 Oct 15. Published in final edited form as: Osteoporos Int. 2004 Jul; 15(7): 552–559.

30. *Br J Nutr*. 2009 Apr;101(8):1113-31. 2008 Oct 1. "Vitamins and Cardiovascular Disease." Honarbakhsh, S., Schachter, M.

31. *Nutr Cancer.* 2009;61(6):767-74. doi: 10.1080/01635580903285155. "Beta-carotene and Lung Cancer in Smokers: Review of Hypotheses and Status of Research." Goralczyk, R.

32. Victor Navarro, et al. "Liver Injury from Herbal and Dietary Supplements." *Hepatology,* Jan. 2017; 65 (1): 363–373.

33. https://www.ncbi.nlm.nih.gov/pmc/articles/PMC5502701/. "Albert Szent-Gyorgyi's Discovery of Vitamin C: International Historic Chemical Landmark." https://www.acs.org/content/acs/en/education/ whatischemistry/landmarks/szentgyorgyi.html.

34. Healthline.com. https://www.healthline.com/nutrition/vitamin-c-deficiency-symptoms.

35. Nutrients. 2017 Mar 29;9(4). pii: E339. doi: 10.3390/nu9040339.

36. Mar 11, 2013 "Ascorbic Acid Supplements and Kidney Stone Incidence Among Men: A Prospective Study." Laura D. K. Thomas, MSc; Carl-Gustaf Elinder, MD; Hans-Göran Tiselius, MD; et al. Alicja Wolk, Dr MedSc; Agneta Åkesson, PhD. *JAMA Intern Med.* 2013;173(5):386-388.

37. Healthline.com. https://www.healthline.com/health/iron-deficiency-anemia.

38. Medpage Today.com. https://www.medpagetoday.com/resource-centers/ focus-on-iron-deficiency-anemia/update-prevalence-causes-and-use-interventions-anemia-worldwide/1648.

39. WebMD.com. https://www.webmd.com/diet/iron-rich-foods#1.

40. Healthline.com. https://www.healthline.com/health/iron-deficiency-anemia#symptoms.

41. MerckManuals.com. https://www.merckmanuals.com/home/hormonal-and-metabolic-disorders/electrolyte-balance/hypomagnesemia-low-level-of-magnesium-in-the-blood.

42. Cedars Mt. Sinai. https://www.cedars-sinai.edu/Patients/Programs-and-Services/Documents/CP0403MagnesiumRichFoods.pdf.

43. Healthline.com. https://www.healthline.com/nutrition/7-common-nutrient-deficiencies#section2sufficient.

44. Ronksley, P.E., Brien, S.E., Turner BJ, et al. "Association of Alcohol Consumption with Selected Cardiovascular Disease Outcomes: A Systematic Review and Meta-Analysis." *BMJ* 2011; 342:d671.

45. "Alcohol and Cardiovascular Health: The Razor-Sharp Double-Edged Sword." O'Keefe, J.H., Bybee, K.A., Lavie, C.J. *J Am Coll Cardiol.* 2007;50(11):1009.

46. "Light to Moderate Intake of Alcohol, Drinking Patterns, and Risk of Cancer: Results from Two Prospective US Cohort Studies." Cao, Y., Willett, W.C., Rimm, E.B., Stampfer, M.J., Giovannucci, E.L. *BMJ*. 2015;351:h4238. Epub 2015 Aug 18.

47. https://www.ncbi.nlm.nih.gov/pmc/articles/PMC5354621/. "The Treasure Called Antibiotics." *Annals of Ibadan Postgraduate Medicine*. W.A. Adedeji, Editor-in-Chief.

48. National Vital Statistics Reports Volume 63, Number 1. "Primary Cesarean Delivery Rates, by State: Results from the Revised Birth Certificate, 2006–2012." by Michelle, J.K. Osterman, M.H.S., and Joyce A. Martin, M.P.H., Division of Vital Statistics.

49. Rebelo, F., da Rocha, C.M., Cortes, T.R., et al. "High Cesarean Prevalence In A National Population-Based Study in Brazil: The Role of Private Practice. *Acta Obstet Gynecol Scand*. 2010;89(7):903–8.

50. *Clin Perinatol*. Author manuscript; available in PMC 2012 Jun 1. Published in final edited form as: *Clin Perinatol*. 2011 Jun; 38(2): 321–331. doi: 10.1016/j.clp.2011.03.008.

51. Strachan, D.P. "Hay Fever, Hygiene, and Household Size." *BMJ*. 1989;299(6710):1259–60. Clin Exp Immunol. 2010 Apr; 160(1): 1–9.

52. "The 'Hygiene Hypothesis' for Autoimmune and Allergic Diseases: An Update. H. Okada, C. Kuhn, H. Feillet, and J.F. Bach.

53. *Environ Health Perspect*. 2008 Mar; 116(3): 303–307. Published online 2007 Dec 7. doi: 10.1289/ehp.10768. "Urinary Concentrations of Triclosan in the U.S. Population: 2003–2004." Antonia M. Calafat, Xiaoyun Ye, Lee-Yang Wong, John A. Reidy, and Larry L. Needham.

54. *Pediatrics*. 2017 Nov;140(Suppl 2):S62-S66. doi: 10.1542/peds.2016-1758D. "Media Multitasking and Cognitive, Psychological, Neural, and Learning Differences." Uncapher, M.R., Lin, L., Rosen, L.D., Kirkorian H.L., Baron, N.S., Bailey, K., Cantor, J., Strayer, D.L., Parsons, T.D., Wagner, A.D.

55. *J Am Heart Assoc*. 2017 Sep 28;6(10). "Meditation and Cardiovascular Risk Reduction: A Scientific Statement From the American Heart Association." Levine, G.N., Lange R.A., Bairey-Merz, C.N., Davidson, R.J., Jamerson, K., Mehta, P.K., Michos E.D., Norris, K., Ray, I.B., Saban, K.L., Shah, T., Stein, R., Smith, S.C. Jr; American Heart Association Council on Clinical Cardiology; Council on Cardiovascular and Stroke Nursing; and Council on Hypertension.

56. *"Meditation Smartphone Application Effects on Prehypertensive Adults' Blood Pressure: Dose-Response Feasibility Trial."* Adams, Z.W., Sieverdes

J.C., Brunner-Jackson B., Mueller, M., Chandler, J., Diaz, V., Patel, S, Sox, L.R., Wilder, S., Treiber, F.A.

57. *J Alzheimers Dis.* 2015;48(1):1-12. doi: 10.3233/JAD-142766. "Stress, Meditation, and Alzheimer's Disease Prevention: Where the Evidence Stands." Khalsa DS1,2.

58. IEEE Signal Process Mag. Author manuscript; available in PMC 2010 Sep 23. IEEE Signal Process Mag. 2008 Jan 1; 25(1): 176–174. *Buddha's Brain: Neuroplasticity and Meditation.* Richard J. Davidson, Director and Antoine Lutz, Associate Scientist.

59. "An update on the pharmacotherapy of attention-deficit/hyperactivity disorder in adults." Wilens, T.E., Morrison, N.R., Prince, J. *Expert Rev Neurother.* 2011;11(10):1443.

60. "Stimulant Medications and Sleep for Youth with ADHD: A Meta-Analysis." Kidwell, K.M., Van Dyk, T.R., Lundahl, A., Nelson, T.D. *Pediatrics.* 2015;136(6):1144.

61. "Long-Term Safety and Efficacy of Lisdexamfetamine Dimesylate in Children and Adolescents with ADHD: A Phase IV, 2-Year, Open-Label Study in Europe." Coghill, D.R., Banaschewski, T., Nagy, P., Otero, I.H., Soutullo, C., Yan, B., Caballero, B., Zuddas, A. CNS Drugs. 2017;31(7):625.

62. "Methylphenidate for Attention Deficit Hyperactivity Disorder (ADHD) in Children and Adolescents: Assessment of Adverse Events in Non-Randomised Studies." StorebøOJ, Pedersen, N., Ramstad, E., Kielsholm, M.L., Nielsen, S.S., Krogh, H.B., Moreira-Maia, C.R., Magnusson, F.L., Holmskov, M., Gerner, T., Skoog, M., Rosendal, S., Groth, C., Gillies, D., Buch Rasmussen, K., Gauci, D., Zwi, M., Kirubakaran, R., Håkonsen, S.J., Aagaard, L., Simonsen, E., Gluud, C. Cochrane Database Syst Rev. 2018;5:CD012069. Epub 2018 May 9.

63. *Am J Public Health.* 2008 June; 98(6): 974–985. "America's First Amphetamine Epidemic 1929–1971: A Quantitative and Qualitative Retrospective with Implications for the Present." Nicolas Rasmussen, PhD, MPhil, MPH.

64. *Exp Clin Psychopharmacol.* 2016 Oct; 24(5): 400–414. "Prescription Stimulant Medication Misuse: Where Are We and Where Do We Go from Here?" Lisa L. Weyandt, PhD, NCSP, Danielle R. Oster, MA, Marisa Ellen Marraccini, PhD, Bergljot Gyda Gudmundsdottir, PhD, Bailey A. Munro, PhD, Emma S. Rathkey, MA, and Alison Mccallum, BS.

65. *Dtsch Arztebl Int.* 2017 Mar; 114(9): 139–141. Published online 2017 Mar 3. "The Natural Course and Treatment of ADHD, and Its Place in Adulthood." Ingrid Schubert, Dr. rer. soc.1, and Gerd Lehmkuhl, em. Prof. Dr. med.2.

66. *Scientific American* Mind (MENTAL HEALTH archives. "The Rise of All-Purpose Antidepressants." Doctors are increasingly prescribing SSRIs to treat more than just depression. By Julia Calderone, November 1, 2014.

67. NCHS Data Brief. 2011 Oct;(76):1-8. "Antidepressant Use in Persons Aged 12 and Over: United States, 2005-2008." Pratt, L.A., Brody, D.J., Gu, Q.

68. Home / *Current Pharmaceutical Design*, Volume 15, Number 14. "Monoaminergic Neurotransmission: The History of the Discovery of Antidepressants from 1950s Until Today." Authors: Lopez-Munoz, Francisco; Alamo, Cecilio. Source: Current Pharmaceutical Design, Volume 15, Number 14, May 2009, pp. 1563-1586(24). Publisher: Bentham Science Publishers.

69. Mayo Clinic Staff. (2016, June 28). Depression (major depressive disorder): "Tricyclic Antidepressants and Tetracyclic Antidepressants." mayoclinic. org/diseases-conditions/depression/in-depth/antidepressants/ART-20046983.

70. Nelson, J.C. "Tricyclic and Tetracyclic Drugs." In: *The American Psychiatric Publishing Textbook of Psychopharmacology*, 4th ed, Schatzberg, AF, Nemeroff, CB (Eds), American Psychiatric Publishing, Washington, DC 2009. P.263.

71. Zahajszky, J, Rosenbaum, et al. Fluoxetine. In: *The American Psychiatric Publishing Textbook of Psychopharmacology*, 4th ed, American Psychiatric Publishing, Inc, Washington, DC 2009. P.289.

72. Labbate, L.A., Fava, et al. "Drugs for the Treatment of Depression." In: *Handbook of Psychiatric Drug Therapy*, 6th ed, Lippincott Williams & Wilkins, Philadelphia, PA 2010. P.54.

73. Ibid. Labbate, et al.

74. "Antidepressant Discontinuation Syndrome." Warner, C.H., Bobo, W., Warner, C., Reid, S., Rachal, J. *Am Fam Physician*. 2006;74(3):449.

75. National Institute for Health and Care Excellence (NICE). *Depression: The Treatment and Management of Depression in Adults* (Updated Edition). Clinical Guideline 90. October, 2009. http://www.nice.org.uk/guidance/cg90 (Accessed on November 06, 2015).

76. "Acid Suppression: Optimizing Therapy for Gastroduodenal Ulcer Healing, Gastroesophageal Reflux Disease, and Stress-Related Erosive Syndrome." Wolfe MM, Sachs G. Gastroenterology. 2000;118(2 Suppl 1):S9. Section of Gastroenterology, Boston University School of Medicine and Boston Medical Center, Massachusetts 02118-2393, USA. micheal.wolfe@bmc.org.

77. "Omeprazole. Overview and Opinion." Holt, S., Howden, C.W. Dig Dis Sci. 1991;36(4):385.

78. "Life Expectancy and Cancer Risk in Patients with Barrett's Esophagus: A Prospective Controlled Investigation." Eckardt, V.F. Kanzler, G., Bernhard, G. *Am J Med*. 2001;111(1):33.

79. "Effects of Proton Pump Inhibitors on Calcium Carbonate Absorption in Women: A Randomized Crossover Trial." O'Connell, M.B., Madden, D.M., Murray, A.M., Heaney, R.P., Kerzner, L.J., *Am J Med*. 2005;118(7):778.

80. "Long-Term Proton Pump Inhibitor Therapy and Risk of Hip Fracture." Yang, Y.X., Lewis, J.D., Epstein, S., Metz, D.C. *JAMA*. 2006;296(24):2947.

81. "Fracture Risk in Patients Receiving Acid-Suppressant Medication Alone and In Combination with Bisphosphonates." de Vries, F., Cooper, A.L., Cockle, S.M., van Staa, T.P., Cooper, C. Osteoporos Int. 2009;20(12):1989. Epub 2009 Mar 3.

82. Hess, M.W., Hoenderop, J.G., Bindels, R.J., et al. "Systematic Review: "Hypomagnesaemia Induced by Proton Pump Inhibition." *Aliment Pharmacol Ther* 2012;36:405–41.

83. Compare, D., Pica, L., Rocco, A., et al. "Effects of Long-Term PPI. Treatment on Producing Bowel Symptoms and SIBO." *Eur J Clin*.

84. *Clinical Gastroenterology and Hepatology* 2013;11:458–464. Perspectives in Clinical Gastroenterology and Hepatology. "Reported Side Effects and Complications of Long-Term Proton Pump Inhibitor Use: Dissecting the Evidence." David A. Johnson and Edward C. Oldfield IV.

85. "Proton Pump Inhibitor Therapy Use Does Not Predispose to Small Intestinal Bacterial Overgrowth." *Am J Gastroenterol* 2012;107:730 –735. Ratuapli SK, Ellington TG, O'Neill MT, et al.

86. "Association of Proton Pump Inhibitors with Risk of Dementia: A Pharmacoepidemiological Claims Data Analysis." Willy Gomm, PhD[1]; Klaus von Holt, MD, PhD; Friederike Thomé, MSc; et al. Karl Broich, MD; Wolfgang Maier, MD; Anne Fink, MSc; Gabriele Doblhammer, PhD; Britta Haenisch, PhD. Author Affiliations Article Information. *JAMA Neurol*. 2016;73(4):410-416.

87. Merlin, M. D. (January 1, 2003). "Archaeological Evidence for the Tradition of Psychoactive Plant Use in the Old World," *Economic Botany*.

88. Paul L. Schiff, Jr., "Opium and its Alkaloids," *American Journal of Pharmaceutical Education*, Summer 2002.

89. Imperial College London Chemical Engineering KKH Research Group website. "Opium, Morphine, and Heroin." Accessed 1.22. 2019. https://www.ch.ic.ac.uk/rzepa/mim/drugs/html/morphine_text.htm.

90. Karolina Brook, Jessica Bennett, Sukumar Desai, "The Chemical History of Morphine: An 8,000-year Hourney, from Resin to denovo Synthesis." *Journal of Anesthesia History*, Volume 3, Issue 2, April 2017.

91. "Opium," from Wikipedia. https://en.wikipedia.org/wiki/ Opium#Recreational_use_in_Europe,_the_Middle_East_and_the_US_ (11th_to_19th_centuries).

92. Journal of the Civil War Era.org. https://www.journalofthecivilwarera. org/2016/11/civil-war-veterans-. Accessed 12. 12, 2019.

93. David T. Courtwright, "The Hidden Epidemic: Opiate Addiction and Cocaine Use in the South, 1860–1920," *The Journal of Southern History 49, no. 1* (February 1988), 83. (Note: information about addicts during the Civil War is also cited in Horace B. Day, *The Opium Habit* (New York: Harper & Brothers, 1868), 6–7) and in an article "Opium and its Consumers," *New York Tribune*, July 10, 1877.

94. David T. Courtwright, *Dark Paradise: A History of Opiate Addiction in America* (Cambridge, Mass: Harvard University Press, 2001).

95. Imperial College London Chemical Engineering KKH Research Group https://www.ch.ic.ac.uk/rzepa/mim/drugs/html/morphine_text.htm. Accessed 1.13, 2019.

96. "Merck Group," Wikipedia. https://en.wikipedia.org/wiki/Merck_Group.

97. Imperial College London Chemical Engineering KKH Research Group. https://www.ch.ic.ac.uk/rzepa/mim/drugs/html/morphine_text.htm. Accessed 1.13. 2019.

98. Addiction Center.com. https://www.addictioncenter.com/opiates/codeine/. Accessed 1.13. 2019.

99. "Oxycodone" from Wikipedia. https://en.wikipedia.org/wiki/Oxycodone

100. "Opium" from Wikipedia. https://en.wikipedia.org/wiki/Opium#cite_ note-9.

101. https://aforeverrecovery.com/blog/information/facts-know-history- oxycodone/.

102. "OxyContin Addiction Facts & Long Term Treatment," The Burning Tree. com. https://www.burningtree.com/oxycontin-addiction/ Acessed 1.12.2019.

103. Max, M.B. "Improving Outcomes Of Analgesic Treatment: Is Education Enough?" *Ann Intern Med*. 1990 Dec 1;113(11):885-9.)

104. The Joint Commission's original standards established in 2001 in an effort to address pain management.

105. Anesth Analg. 2005 Jan;100(1):162-8. "The Impact of The Joint Commission For Accreditation Of Healthcare Organizations Pain Initiative on Perioperative Opiate Consumption and Recovery Room Length of Stay." Frasco PE1, Sprung J, Trentman TL.

106. "The Joint Commission's Pain Standard: Origins and Evolution" by David Baker MD, MPH, Executive VP Division of Healthcare Quality Evaluation May 5, 2017.

107. National Institute on Drug Abuse. "America's Addiction to Opioids: Heroin and Prescription Drug Abuse." May 14, 2014. *presented by* Nora D. Volkow, MD., Senate Caucus on International Narcotics Control.

108. *Am J Public Health.* 2009 February; 99(2): 221–227. "The Promotion and Marketing of OxyContin: Commercial Triumph, Public Health Tragedy." Art Van Zee, MD.

109. Anesthesia Clinics. "Advancing the Pain Agenda in the Veteran Population." By Rollin Gallagher, MD MPH. June 2016 Volume 34, Issue 2, Pages 357–378.

110. An Official Website of the Department of Veterans Affairs. US Department of Veterans Affairs. Department of Veteran Affairs Opioid Prescribing Data.

111. "Guide to the Female Reproductive System," WebMD Medical Reference. https://www.webmd.com/menopause/qa/how-many-eggs-does-a-woman-have.

112. "Risk of Endometrial Cancer Following Estrogen Replacement with and without Progestins." Elisabete Weiderpass, Hans-Olov Adami, John A. Baron, Cecilia Magnusson, Reinhold Bergström, Anders Lindgren, Nestor Correia, Ingemar Persson. *JNCI: Journal of the National Cancer Institute,* Volume 91, Issue 13, 7 July 1999, Pages 1131–1137.

113. *Clinical Cancer Research* "Estrogen, Estrogen Plus Progestin Therapy, and Risk of Breast Cancer." Graham A. Colditz. January 2005. Volume 11, Issue 2.

114. *New England Journal of Medicine.* "Estrogen and the Risk of Breast Cancer." Mark Clemons, M.B., B.S., M.D., and Paul Goss, M.D., Ph.D. January 25, 2001. N Engl J Med 2001; 344:276-285.

115. Evening Use of Light-Emitting Ereaders Negatively Affects Sleep, Circadian Timing, and Next-Morning Alertness. Chang, A.M., Aeschbach, D., Duffy, J.F., Czeisler, C.A. *Proc Natl Acad Sci USA.* 2015;112(4):1232. Epub 2014 Dec 22.

116. "Increased Physical Activity Improves Sleep and Mood Outcomes in Inactive People with Insomnia: A Randomized Controlled Trial." Hartescu, I., Morgan, K., Stevinson, C.D. *J Sleep Res.* 2015 Oct;24(5):526-34. Epub 2015 Apr 21.

117. "You and Your Hormones."An Educational Resource from the Society for Endocrinology. www.yourhormones.info/hormones/melatonin/.

118. "Fall in Nocturnal Serum Melatonin During Prepuberty and Pubescence." Waldhauser, F., Weiszenbacher, G., Frisch, H., Zeitlhuber, U., Waldhauser, M., Wurtman, R.J. *Lancet.* 1984;1(8373):362.

119. "Melatonin Desensitizes Endogenous MT2 Melatonin Receptors in the Rat Suprachiasmatic Nucleus: Relevance for Defining the Periods of Sensitivity of the Mammalian Circadian Clock to Melatonin." Gerdin, M.J., Masana, M.I., Rivera-Bermúdez, M.A., Hudson, R.L., Earnest, D.J., Gillette, M.U., Dubocovich, M.L. *FASEB J.* 2004;18(14):1646.

120. "Melatonin-Mediated Regulation Of Human MT(1) Melatonin Receptors Expressed In Mammalian Cells." Gerdin, M.J., Masana, M.I., Dubocovich, M.L. *Biochem Pharmacol.* 2004;67(11):2023.

121. "Safety in Melatonin Use." Morera, A.L., Henry, M., de La Varga, M. *Actas Esp Psiquiatr.* 2001;29(5):334.

122. March 2015. "Cumulative Use of Strong Anticholinergics and Incident Dementia A Prospective Cohort Study." Shelly L. Gray, PharmD, MS; Melissa L. Anderson, MS; Sascha Dublin, MD, PhD; et al. Joseph T. Hanlon, PharmD, MS; Rebecca Hubbard, PhD; Rod Walker, MS; Onchee Yu, MS; Paul K. Crane, MD, MPH; Eric B. Larson, MD, MPH.

123. UpToDate.com. "Overview of the Treatment of Insomnia in Adults." Author: John W Winkelman, MD, PhD; Section Editor: Ruth Benca, MD, PhD; Deputy Editor: April F Eichler, MD, MPH. Accessed Jan. 18, 2019.

124. "Environmental Pollutants and Disease In American Children: Estimates of Morbidity, Mortality, and Costs for Lead Poisoning, Asthma, Cancer, and Developmental Disabilities. Landrigan, P.J., Schechter, C.B., Lipton, J.M., Fahs, M.C., Schwartz, J. *Environ Health Perspect.* 2002;110(7):721.

125. "Occupational Asthma." Tarlo, S.M., Lemiere, C. *N Engl J Med.* 2014 Feb;370(7):640-9.

126. "An Official American Thoracic Society Statement: Work-Exacerbated Asthma." Henneberger, P.K., Redlich, C.A., Callahan, D.B., Harber, P., Lemière, C., Martin, J., Tarlo, S.M., Vandenplas, O., Torén, K. ATS Ad Hoc Committee on Work-Exacerbated Asthma. *Am J Respir Crit Care Med.* 2011;184(3):368.

127. "An Association Between Air Pollution and Mortality in Six U.S. Cities." Dockery, D.W., Pope, C.A., 3rd, Xu X, Spengler, J.D., Ware, J.H., Fay, M.E., Ferris, B.G., Jr, Speizer, F.E. *N Engl J Med*. 1993;329(24):1753.

128. Main Air Pollutants and Myocardial Infarction: A Systematic Review and Meta-Analysis. Mustafic, H., Jabre, P., Caussin, C., Murad, M.H., Escolano, S., Tafflet, M., Périer, M.C., Marijon, E., Vernerey, D., Empana, J.P. *Jouven X JAMA*. 2012;307(7):713.

129. Byeong-Jae Kee, et al. "Air Pollution Exposure and Cardiovascular Disease." https://www.ncbi.nlm.nih.gov/pmc/articles/PMC4112067/.

130. Ibid.

131. "Montreal Protocol" essay on Wikipedia. https://en.wikipedia.org/wiki/Montreal_Protocol.

132. "Radon in Homes and Risk of Lung Cancer: Collaborative Analysis of Individual Data from 13 European Case-Control Studies." Darby, S., Hill, D., Auvinen, A., Barros-Dios, J.M., Baysson, H., Bochicchio, F., Deo, H., Falk, R., Forastiere, F., Hakama, M., Heid, I., Kreienbrock, L., Kreuzer, M., Lagarde, F., Mäkeläinen, I., Muirhead, C., Oberaigner, W., Pershagen, G., Ruano-Ravina, A., Ruosteenoja, E., Rosario, A.S., Tirmarche, M., Tomásek, L., Whitley, E., Wichmann, H.E., Doll, R. *BMJ*. 2005;330(7485):223. Epub 2004 Dec 21.

133. *Front Neurosci*. 2018 Aug 30;12:612. doi: 10.3389/fnins.2018.00612. eCollection 2018. "Parkinson's Disease: Biomarkers, Treatment, and Risk Factors." Emamzadeh, F.N., Surguchov, A.

134. *Toxicol Sci*. 2018 Sep 7. "Inflammasomes: An Emerging Mechanism Translating Environmental Toxicant Exposure into Neuroinflammation in Parkinson's Disease." Anderson, F.L., Coffey, M.M., Berwin, B.L., Havrda, M.C.

135. Swaminathan, K. "Pesticides and Human Diabetes: A Link Worth Exploring?" *Diabet Med*. 2013 Nov;30(11):1268-71. doi: 10.1111/dme.12212.

136. BMC Public Health. 2017 June 28;17(1):602. "Childhood Pesticide Poisoning in Zhejiang, China: A Retrospective Analysis from 2006 to 2015." Yimaer, A., Chen, G., Zhang, M., Zhou, L., Fang, X., Jiang, W.

137. "Low Level Methylmercury Exposure Affects Neuropsychological Function in Adults." Yokoo, E.M., Valente, J.G., Grattan, L., Schmidt, S.L., Platt, I., Silbergeld, E.K.. *Environ Health*. 2003 Jun;2(1):8. Epub 2003 Jun 4.

138. "Thimerosal in Vaccines," Centers for Diease Controland Prevention: Vaccine Safety https://www.cdc.gov/vaccinesafety/concerns/thimerosal/index.html. Accessed 1.22. 2019.

139. "Thimerosal and Vaccines," U.S. Food & Drug Administration. https://www.fda.gov/BiologicsBloodVaccines/SafetyAvailability/VaccineSafety/UCM096228. Accessed 1.22.2019.

140. Brian Koberstein, "Why Anti-Vaxxers Are Wrong About Methyl Mercury in Shots, Forbes.com. https://www.forbes.com/sites/briankoberlein/2016/09/20/vaccines-meteors-and-why-details-matter/#6d4090d91939.

141. Wakefield, A., Murch, S., Anthony, A., et al. (1998). "Ileal-Lymphoid-Nodular Hyperplasia, Non-Specific Colitis, and Pervasive Developmental Disorder in Children." *Lancet.* 351(9103): 637–641. doi:10.1016/S0140-6736(97)11096-0. PMID 9500320. Retrieved 2007-09-05. (Retracted)

142. *The Lancet.* Volume 353, Issue 9169, 12 June 1999, pages 2026-2029. "Autism and Measles, Mumps, and Rubella Vaccine: No Epidemiological Evidence for a Causal Association." Prof. Brent Taylor, FRCP, Chair Elizabeth Miller, FRCPath, Paddy Farrington, PhD, Maria-Christina Petropoulos, MRCP, Isabelle Favot-Mayaud, MD., Jun Li, PhD, Pauline A. Waight, BS cb.

143. "Andrew Wakefield" article from Wikipedia; https://en.wikipedia.org/wiki/Andrew_Wakefield.

144. Kaye, J.A., del Mar Melero-Montes, M., Jick, H. "Mumps, Measles, and Rubella Vaccine and yhe Incidence of Autism Recorded by General Practitioners: A Time Trend Analysis." *BMJ.* 2001;322:460–3.Deer B (2004-02-22). "Revealed: MMR research scandal." *The Sunday Times.* Retrieved 2007-09-23.

Index

N

About the Author

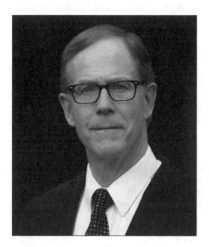

STEPHEN C. BREWER, MD, ABFM, is the Medical Director at Canyon Ranch Wellness Resorts in Tucson, Arizona. He was an associate fellow in the Integrative Medicine Program at the University of Arizona where he studied under the direction of Dr. Andrew Weil. He was trained and certified in acupuncture at UCLA and is certified in guided imagery. He received his medical degree from the Medical College of Ohio, completed his residency in Family Medicine at Riverside Methodist Hospital, and is board certified in Family Medicine. He has been practicing medicine for over thirty-five years. Dr. Brewer started his medical career as a country doctor and then later became an assistant director of a family medicine residency. He was the first medical director of Integrative medicine at the Trihealth Hospital system in Cincinnati, Ohio. His areas of special expertise include family medicine, integrative medicine, medical acupuncture, fibromyalgia, central sensitization, preventative medicine and men's health.

Dr. Brewer is the author of the book *The Canyon Ranch Guide to Men's Health* published in 2016 and coauthored *The Everest Principle: How to Achieve the Summit of Your Life* in 2010. He wrote a chapter on men's health in the book, *Integrative Preventive Medicine* and helped in the writing of the book, *30 Days to a Better Brain*. He has published journal articles that include: "Cognitive Loss in Later life: The Challenge for Family and Community" written for *The Journal on Active Aging*. He has on-line pieces, including "Acupuncture for Athletes: Sticking It to Injuries" and "Peak Performance and Sleep"published on active.com and coauthored a piece for Maria Shriver's annual Women's Conference website titled "The Everest Principle or How to Reach Your Peak Performance." He was a keynote speaker for several events that include Saint Lucia's Wellness Conference in 2011 and 2012 and the University of Arizona College of medicine event on "Living Healthy with Arthritis." Dr. Brewer has also given medical grand rounds at Mayo Clinic in Scottsdale, Albany Medical School in New York, and at the University of Arizona Department of Integrative Medicine.